MENOPAUSE

CHANGE, CHOICE AND HRT

DR BARRY G. WREN

MARGARET STEPHENSON MEERE

ROCKPOOL PUBLISHING

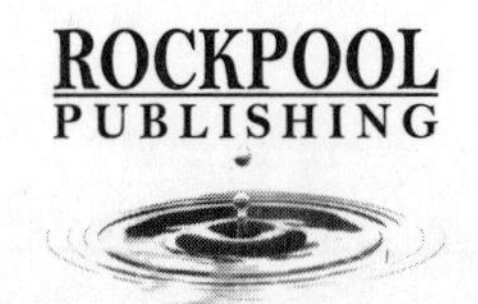

A Rockpool book
PO Box 252
Summer Hill
NSW 2130
Australia
www.rockpoolpublishing.com.au
http://www.facebook.com/RockpoolPublishing

First published in 2013

National Library of Australia Cataloguing-in-Publication entry

Wren, Barry G. (Barry George)
Menopause: change, choice and hrt
Dr Barry Wren; Margaret Stephenson Meere.
978 1 9218 7869 5 (pbk.)
Includes index.
Menopause.
Menopause–Treatment.
Menopause–Alternative treatment.
Menopause–Hormone therapy.
618.175

Cover design by Ingrid Kwong
Edited by Jody Lee
Illustrations by Swift Prosys
Typeset by Peter Guo, Letterspaced
Printed and bound in India by Replika Press Pvt. Ltd.

10 9 8 7 6 5 4 3 2

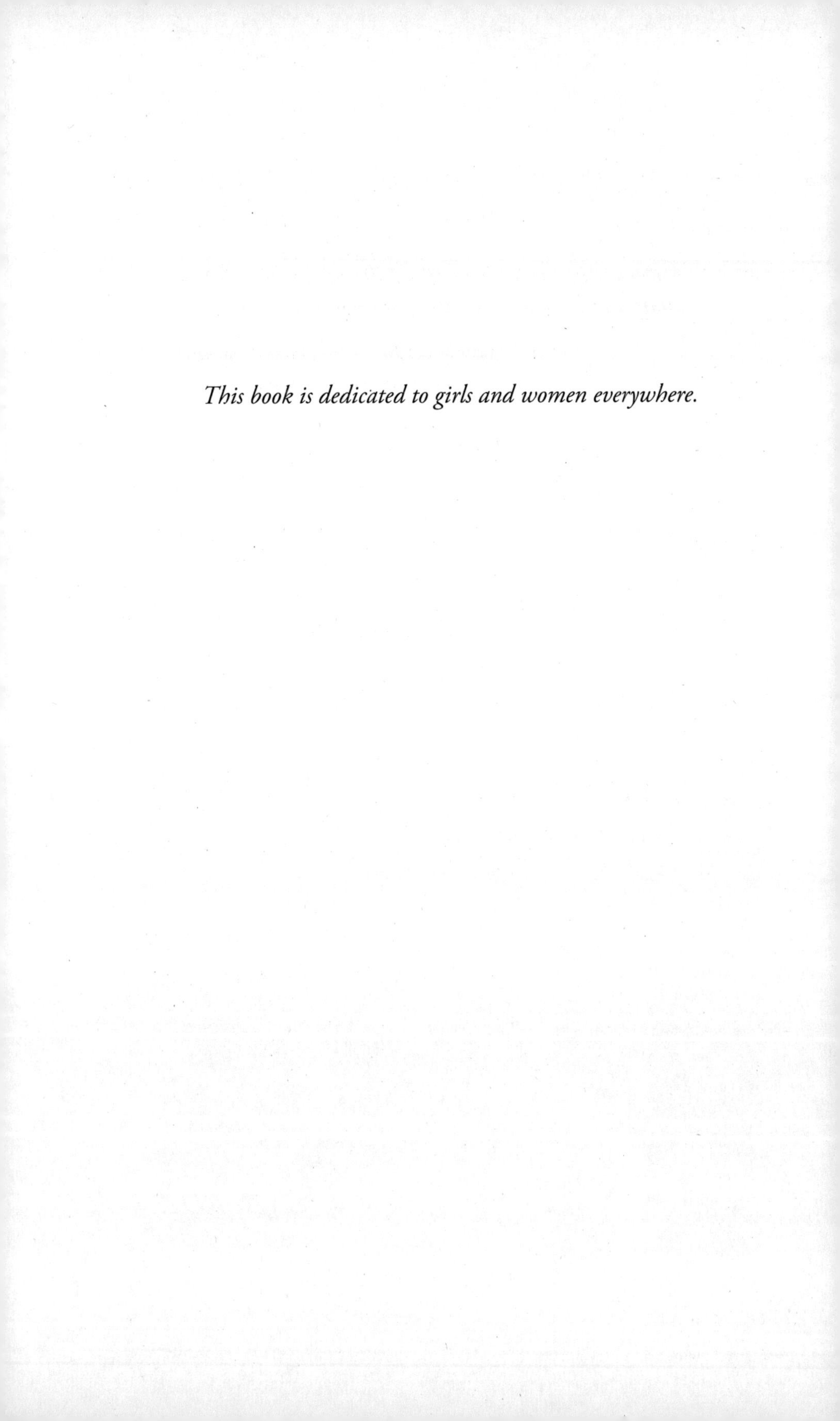

This book is dedicated to girls and women everywhere.

A woman in the autumn of her life deserves an Indian summer rather than a winter of discontent.

— Robert Greenblatt, 1907–1987, First President,
International Menopause Society

To everything there is a season, and a time to every purpose under the heaven:

a time to be born and a time to die;

a time to plant, and a time to pluck up that which is planted;

a time to kill, and a time to heal;

a time to break down, and a time to build up;

a time to weep, and a time to laugh;

a time to mourn and a time to dance;

a time to cast away stones, and a time to gather stones together;

a time to embrace, and a time to refrain from embracing;

a time to get, and a time to lose;

a time to keep, and a time to cast away;

a time to rend, and a time to sew;

a time to keep silence, and a time to speak;

a time to love, and a time to hate;

a time of war, and a time of peace.

— Ecclesiastes 3:1-8, *The Book of Wisdom*

How to use this book

This book has been written for women, to explain the menopause and the influence of the ovary and its hormones on a woman's body and health. It is a guide to help them make choices for their future health and life potential. This is not a book that needs to be read from beginning to end, nor is it a book of hard science. It is a book written to explain the history, biology, scientific studies and treatments for the menopause, a time in a woman's life that has until now, been a mystery and often a misery for many.

While this book has been created primarily for women, it has been structured in a way that makes it accessible for all readers. Consequently it has been divided into five sections for quick access to the essence of its content. The first four sections cover the history and definition of menopause and Hormone Replacement Therapy (HRT), menopause and health, the management of menopause, and finally the therapy choices or options that are available.

For the reader who scans the book there are the summaries that conclude each chapter in the first three sections. For the reader who wants to probe more widely, there is extensive detailed information in the body of each chapter. The fourth section of the book provides an overview of menopause today. Section five contains the appendices for the reader who wants to delve more deeply into the many different therapies of the menopause as well as providing more details of hormones and cancer.

Menopause is a time in every woman's life that is a journey of personal change and new growth. This journey does not come with a road map. However, this book provides some direction and new understanding of the menopause. It is up to a woman herself to choose her own path, and to determine how she wants to achieve her intended purpose in life.

Author's note

In my practice as a gynaecologist, I ask a woman attending her first consultation to complete a short questionnaire. This provides me with her relevant essential personal details and helps me to ascertain what she perceives to be her concerns or problems. At the end of the questionnaire there are a few lines available for comments or questions that she may have. These comments and enquiries contain some of the most enlightening statements regarding the impact the menopause may have on a woman. Among the hundreds of written comments, the most frequent are those expressing confusion and bewilderment. The questions most often asked are 'How long does the menopause last?', 'Why do I feel so flat?', 'I've lost interest in everything – is this due to the menopause?', 'Can I do something to prevent my body from deteriorating?', 'What can I do to prevent osteoporotic fractures?', 'Is it alright to have sex?', 'Will I be able to have a satisfactory relationship with a new sexual partner?', 'If I begin hormone therapy, can I fall pregnant?', 'Will I go mad/demented if I take HRT?', 'Will I be able to do the things I did before the change?', 'What will become of me?', 'What can I do?'

A woman today has a good general knowledge about sex and contraception, and she can readily obtain information on matters such as rearing children and coping with inter-personal family matters. However, the symptoms of her menopause can come as a surprise and the management of them is surrounded in confusion and controversy. The underlying physiology of the menopause is also a mystery for many women. They want to know what is happening to them, how the menopause will affect their future, and what options are available to treat their problems.

It became apparent that the majority of women attending my office had no clear idea of the physiology of ovarian hormone activity, the effect of hormone deficiency on cells and organs in the body, or the possible treatment options to reduce the effects of hormone deficiency. They complained that often their busy family doctor diagnosed them as suffering from 'the menopause' but cautioned that hormone treatment caused breast cancer or stroke which meant that hormone replacement therapy was contraindicated. Very few family doctors are able to give the time to discuss the role of hormones in maintaining health and quality of life, or in reducing disease, nor are they able to discuss recent research results related to breast cancer, heart attacks, hypertension, dementia or osteoporosis. Alternative therapies such as neurotransmitter inhibiters, plant extracts, herbal mixes and other treatments are offered as a means of reducing hot flushes, but there is very little or no advice regarding the reduction of other diseases associated with the post-menopause.

For more than 30 years, I have written a number of books for medical students and doctors to provide medical information on hormones and hormone replacement therapy. Some of the women attending my consulting rooms acquired copies of these or other medical books related to the menopause, in order to obtain the information for which they were searching. Most of those who had read my medical books were complimentary about the information and many suggested that I should write a book especially for them – one which would explain the physiology and the long-term effect of hormone deficiency so that all women could understand it and make their own decisions about their available options.

Even though the post-menopause will last for about half of their adult life, women have not been able to easily obtain accurate and unbiased information about the changes that will happen to them during a significant phase of their life.

Many women have criticised their family doctor for not explaining the impact of estradiol and testosterone deficiency as well as the importance and significance of progesterone. Some women have blamed the media for accentuating and exaggerating the adverse findings in the Women's Health Initiative study report, and many have been angry with the media for not providing a balanced and objective coverage of research about the menopause. In presenting the information in this book, I have based all the evidence and information on the many research reports which have been published by scientists working in institutions that have an impeccable reputation. All significant papers from which I have drawn my information are listed in the reference section. In quoting important research and published results, I have attempted to make the details easily understood and, I hope, of value, for women who ask 'why does this happen?'

For all of you who have requested it, here is your book.

BARRY G. WREN

CONTENTS

SECTION THREE

Prologue

In the last few decades, the demographic profile of a woman's life has changed – a young woman is now delaying her entry into commitment with a partner and an opportunity of parenting in order to pursue a career, or to travel the world before what used to be euphemistically called 'settling down'.

She feels she is invincible!

Today, a new mother is often well into her middle to late thirties, or even in her forties when not only is she experiencing the rigours of pregnancy, her birthing process and the raising of very young children, it is also the time when she may be entering her years of peri-menopause. It can be a very challenging time for her and her partner. This sociological change is not generally appreciated because a woman of today is remaining physically and mentally younger in her years with a belief that, as she will live a longer life than her parents with an average life span now of about 84 years, she has plenty of time left for family responsibilities.

However, her ovaries have not yet caught up with this social and scientific evolution (this will take a lot more than just a few thousand years), so even though a woman's physical and mental maturity is developing over a longer span of time, her ovaries and their hormones and eggs begin to decline when she is in her mid to late thirties.

This is a book about hormones, particularly estrogen – what it is, what it does for a woman, and what happens to her when her body stops producing it. Estrogen is what makes a girl into a woman. It is involved in initiating menstruation, having a pregnancy, maintaining her feminine beauty and her vigour and when her ovaries no longer produce it, to mark the completion of her childbearing years. The changes resulting from loss of estrogen are often found to coincide with her years of maturity and freedom and although the symptoms of estrogen deficiency can be distressing, scientific research is revealing that estrogen can alleviate her problems and protect her in her future years.

In her maturity, a woman can determine who she is, and how she wants to live her life. She is responsible for her own health and the choices that she makes for it. The choices she makes in her menopausal years are particularly important.

This book has the strength of two voices – one has the knowledge and experience of a gynaecologist who, for over three decades, has researched the menopause and facilitated many grateful women through it. The other is the voice of a woman who has traversed the years of her menopause, made her choices, and emerged stronger in her new life and career.

There is some technical language in the book, but the science of the human body can't avoid this. It is important for us to know our own self, not only our physical body but also the mental and emotional aspects as well, but this knowledge and the gaining of it requires endeavour and exploration in order to understand who we really are. Knowledge empowers and allows individuals to understand their life, to make decisions for themselves and to manage their own destiny.

Over the last 100 years women, with courage, have emancipated themselves and they continue to do so. However, there is still a way to travel because strangely, even though we are better educated, we are often ignorant of the function of our own body and quite at sea when it comes to how a woman functions physiologically in her middle and older age.

A girl now has a good basic knowledge of her first rite of passage – her menarche – and is better prepared for it through her schooling and a more open home environment. Her next rite of passage is more one of choice – the choosing to have a child – and this journey is well catered for through information in the media and also in pregnancy, childbirth and parenting education programs.

A woman's third rite of passage is not of her choosing. It is the inevitability of her menopause, which still remains a mystery – a silent passage with no celebration, very little understanding and no education. This must change if a woman wants to continue to move forward with the respect and support and growth that is her right.

Up until now, some women have endured a miserable and often confusing period of personal turmoil in their menopause transition that may have lasted for years, as any possibility of dialogue about their menopause has been stifled by their own lack of knowledge of it and a sense of shame and grief for her loss of youth and reproductive capacity. Self-knowledge can help a woman to deal with the grief as well as grant her the courage to gather together with other women to talk about her fears, to learn from others, and to develop an understanding and compassion for other women in their transition.

For too long and, in more ways than one, the menopause has been a silent time in a woman's life. It has been silent because there has existed a belief that it is a 'natural event in a woman's life'; that there was nothing that could or should be done about it; and it has also been silent because it hasn't been privately talked about or publicly debated.

Introduction

When a woman has passed the age of procreation and she is no longer committed to active motherhood, she begins her age of creative energy, independent thought, and freedom of action. She, as a woman of our modern era, now rejects the old notion that she is expected to accept the passive, dutiful or obedient role associated with older age. In spite of her concerns and doubts about her future, she is now able to welcome her post-menopausal years. It is a time that can become a springboard for a new, different and exciting phase in her life. The important issue is – how can a woman cope with 'the change'.

In the year 1900, women in Australia had an average life span of 59 years. While those living beyond 60 years were treated with veneration and respect, most were not expected to remain in, or to maintain a dominant role in society or to be actively involved in community affairs. Now, only 100 years later, their average life expectancy has increased to 84 years and women in the 21st century can expect to live over 40 per cent (35–40 years) of their lives after they have passed the menopause.

The menopause has become a dramatic marker of a change in physiology and body function for all women. Some women may experience severe flushes, sweats, insomnia, mood swings, depression, loss of interest, loss of drive and loss of libido, while others may develop osteoporosis, heart attacks, dementia or cancer.

For hundreds of years, women have traditionally been categorised into three ages – the maiden, the mother and the wise old crone, or matriarch. But the 20th century ushered in the fourth age of a woman – the age of liberation and – an age for development – to be a mentor and adviser, passing on life experiences to younger women, supporting daughters and grandchildren and re-creating themselves with new vigour and determination. She now has the freedom and the years to embark on a new career, and to find new interests – the age to have fun and to enjoy life – the age of re-creation. This fourth age is the age when a woman who, having produced, nurtured and educated her children, and created a home for her family, gains the freedom in which to re-create herself as a significant individual, embarking on a new life, with new choices and the opportunity to develop a new vocation and the freedom to express her new sexuality. It is the age when a woman who, having ventured into one career path in her youth, should be able to receive the acclaim she deserves as she advances in her new chosen profession.

Women (and men) are taking much longer to become 'old'.

However, many women do not enjoy the extra years they are now given – they are often adversely affected by the physical, psychological and sexual changes associated with loss of the hormones that, until the menopause, are produced by the ovary in order to maintain normal function of cells. For a large number of post-menopausal women, the use of sex hormone therapy to maintain activity of dependent cells, may allow them to continue their career, to embark on a new venture, to save their marriage or even begin a new life.

Mary, a woman in her late forties held a very senior position in a government department. She was lauded by her colleagues and political masters as being an exceptional public servant and, as a consequence, had been promoted to head a very important department. She was regarded as not only being an exceptionally intelligent woman but an outstanding administrator.

Then, without warning, she began to experience severe and distressing migraine headaches, episodes of memory disturbance, night sweats and embarrassing hot flushes. She felt her 'brain was made of cotton wool'. These symptoms were so disturbing that she was unable to function adequately in meetings with government ministers and other senior bureaucrats. She often burst into tears for no apparent reason, and suffered extreme mood swings.

She saw her doctor who was concerned about her psychological state and the severity of her symptoms. He referred her to a psychiatrist who prescribed an anti-depressant and a sedative. When after three months there was no improvement, she felt convinced she had a brain tumour and this fear was accentuated by several episodes of panic attacks, insecurity and depression. She was even more devastated when her partner of many years decided he could not cope with her mood swings, outbursts of anger and her irrational behaviour and marked loss of libido. He decided to separate from her. After almost twelve months with no relief from various therapies (mostly psycho-trophic drugs such as anti-depressants, anxiolytic agents and sedatives) prescribed by her doctor, and distressed and embarrassed by her symptoms, she resigned from her position. Because of the marked effect on her general health and her wellbeing, she contemplated suicide.

> Her sister, who was receiving hormone therapy, thought there may be a hormonal problem and persuaded her to attend the clinic at the Menopause Centre at the Royal Hospital for Women in Sydney. Her medical history revealed that she had suffered from severe and painful periods and for that reason a hysterectomy had been performed when she was 32. Physical examination and investigations confirmed that she was markedly deficient in ovarian hormones, so she was advised to begin hormone therapy.
>
> Within a week of having estradiol and testosterone implants inserted in the fat in her lower abdomen she began to feel 'normal' again and her symptoms disappeared. Unfortunately she was unable to resume her previous position with the government. Her expectations of a successful career as the head of her department had been shattered by the onset of her 'menopause'.

Mary's story is not unique. Many women have told of their distress as they have attempted to cope with overwhelming change in their ability to function during and following the time of gradual loss of their ovarian hormones.

The classic image of the menopause is of a woman fanning herself vigorously as she experiences a flush associated with uncontrolled sweating, or it is of an older lady who has a dowager's hump following osteoporotic fractures of her spine.

Loss of estradiol at the menopause is frequently associated with other distressing personal problems such as insomnia, poor verbal memory recall, dementia, psychological or emotional disturbances, increasing urinary frequency, a dry vagina and loss of libido.

During the post-menopause, a woman may continue to suffer from a variety of distressing symptoms such as flushes and sweats, emotional and psychological depression or discomfort during sexual intercourse (sometimes leading to rejection by a partner). She may also develop some disfiguring physical changes (a dowager's hump) or premature skin deterioration (wrinkles, fragile skin) and, because of these changes, she often experiences social humiliation and isolation.

Until the middle of the 20th century, life for many post-menopausal women was bleak and depressing, with little reduction in the progression towards crush fractures of the spine due to osteoporosis with subsequent immobility; memory loss, Alzheimer's dementia, or premature death from heart attacks. Many women continued to experience the peri-menopausal symptoms of distressing flushes, sweats, insomnia and marked sexual problems into their advanced age.

With the availability of relatively cheap commercial quantities of sex hormones (estradiol, progesterone and testosterone) the situation for a woman has changed and she now has access to reliable hormone treatment options.

For all women it is vitally important that the normal function of cells in the brain, bones, muscles, the heart and other vital organs is maintained. There are many therapies, both medical and non-medical, which may help to maintain the vitality of a post-menopausal woman. These include regular exercise, the maintenance of normal weight, the stimulating of brain function with mental exercise programs and to give up smoking.

Hormone therapy can also help with this maintenance. There are hundreds of hormones produced in various glands and organs and all are involved in maintaining and integrating the normal function of the millions of cells in our body. Just as an orchestra is composed of many musicians who work together under the baton of a conductor to play beautiful music, hundreds of hormone messengers are controlled and directed by the hypothalamus of the brain and the pituitary gland to enable the harmonious function of our body. If one musician in the orchestra is out of tune or plays to a different score, it upsets the other players and results in musical discord. If, in the body, the amount of any hormone is inappropriate or insufficient to maintain normal cell function, the body responds with marked changes that disturb the normal body homeostasis or balanced function.

The ovary is the only organ in the human body that is programmed to fail.

From birth onwards there is a steady decline in the number of eggs and their follicles in the ovary until about the age of 40–45 years, when the rate of loss of hormones increases rapidly. All women will experience ovarian hormone deficiency as their ovaries run out of eggs. The years during which the failing ovaries attempt to maintain estrogen production is known as the peri-menopause. It is during this phase of their life, that irregular menstruation, mood swings and menopausal symptoms become obvious even before a woman finally becomes post-menopausal. No two women will experience peri-menopause in the same way nor will they experience it over the same period of time. However, it is during her time in the peri-menopause that a woman will seek out help to understand what she is experiencing and also to determine if there is anything that can be done to alleviate her symptoms.

The introduction and use of hormone therapy has not been without controversy, and has been associated with both medical and societal opposition. For many years, the post-menopause has been regarded as an unwelcome phase in a woman's life. It has been associated with prejudices, negative opinions and often distortion of facts regarding the causes and management of symptoms. Often these menopausal symptoms persisted and became particularly distressing for women who were confronted with deterioration in their energy levels and also their ability to maintain their previous roles in life.

In early China and other parts of Asia, and later in Ancient Greece and Rome, physicians prescribed and used many herbs, fungi, potions and other interventions in an attempt to assist a woman who was experiencing severe symptoms or problems after her menopause. None of these botanical remedies provided permanent or overall relief from the symptoms or the emotional disruptions of the menopause and, as a consequence, many women were regarded in a negative light once they entered their post-menopause.

However, in the late 1930s, a dramatic change in therapy options became available and, since then, hormone replacement therapy has dominated the management of the menopause. For over 70 years, various estrogens and other sex hormones have been used to treat post-menopausal women who complain of hot flushes, sweats, insomnia or a dry vagina; who have memory disturbances, emotional and mood swings, or who have loss of drive, energy and libido. During these years, not only did estrogen improve symptoms and quality of life, it was also observed in many studies and research projects, that a woman who used estrogen had less risk of osteoporotic fractures, heart attacks or dementia than did a woman who was not given this therapy.

Because of such beneficial reports from observational studies, it was decided in 1991 to conduct a prospective randomised controlled trial to determine if hormone therapy could improve the long-term health of a post-menopausal woman and therefore provide a benefit for her.

A huge study, the Women's Health Initiative (WHI) Study was conducted under the auspices of the National Institute of Health in the United States with the intention of determining the health outcome of women as they aged. Initially it involved the recruitment of 161,809 women, aged 50 to 79 years, of whom 27,347 women entered a subgroup, which became the focus of the Hormone Replacement Therapy (HRT) project. At entry, this subgroup of women was randomly allocated to receive either hormone therapy or a placebo.

In 2002, the first paper from the WHI Writing Group reported that hormone therapy, consisting of an estrogen and a progestogen (progestin), was associated with an increased risk of breast cancer, heart attacks, stroke and dementia.[1] As a result of these findings, and the manner of their release, hormone therapy was reported by the media to be an initiator of cancer and cardiovascular disease. Women were urged by hastily convened advisory committees to stop using hormone therapy.

Following the panic and hysteria surrounding the first of what was to be many reports related to the WHI Study, a large number of women stopped hormone therapy and many switched to alternative (natural) treatments that were being offered, in order to relieve the distressing symptoms of the menopause. In spite of intense publicity and advertising campaigns promoting these therapy options, the majority of women who tried first one, then a second or even a third alternative therapy, continued to express disappointment at the failure of these treatment options to relieve symptoms or prevent deterioration in specific hormone dependent parts of their body. Members of the medical profession also expressed concern and scepticism regarding a number of the claims being made for these alternative treatment programs, particularly those which were not based on carefully conducted scientific evidence. Because of the many conflicting assertions, opinions and reports about the merits, advantages and adverse effects of both alternative and regular hormone therapy programs, post-menopausal women and their health advisers have been undecided about which of the various therapies on offer for management of the menopause are examples of 'snake oil', which convey no benefit or might even cause harm, and therapies which are 'good oils' that convey an advantage to those who use them.

In this book the clinical evidence of the effects of hormone deficiency at the menopause is discussed, and information and references regarding the advantages, as well as the imperfections, of frequently prescribed hormones and other medicines that are used to manage the menopause, are presented. This information is offered to help a woman decide which treatment program is most suitable for her during her peri- and post-menopausal years when her symptoms and her failing hormone system interfere with her life, her relationships and her dreams and expectations.

Section One

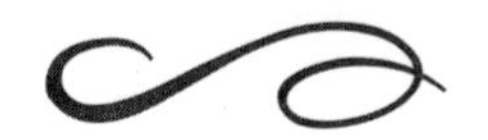

History, Menopause, HRT and the Women's Health Initiative Study

CHAPTER 1

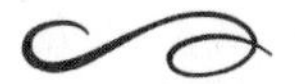

A history of the menopause and HRT

From pre-Christian history to the 19th century, knowledge about a woman's menstrual activity and its causes was dominated by a male perception of how it came about, what its purpose was, and what happened when a woman stopped menstruating. Early Greek and Roman physicians felt that menstrual blood was necessary to rid the female body of 'bad humours' and that the symptoms of the menopause came about because the accumulated toxins in the menstrual blood were not being released.

The biblical description of menstruation and its effect suggests it was regarded with repellence. In Leviticus 15, menstrual discharge is described '*when a woman has a discharge of blood which is her regular discharge from her body, she shall be in her impurity for seven days, and whoever touches her shall be unclean until the evening*'.

Early education regarding menstruation was taught by monks and philosophers as they were the only people in the community who could read or write. One group of monks inhabiting northern Britain was responsible for *The Aberdeen Bestiary* written in the 12th century. It was their understanding of the physiology of animals, birds and flora, and the following is a description by these monks of their understanding of menstruation.

'The menstrual flow is the superfluous blood of a woman. It is called menstrua from the cycle of the light of the moon, which regularly brings about this flow. For the Greek word for "moon" is mene; menstruation is also called muliebria, "womanly business". For the woman is the only creature which menstruates. When they come into contact with menstrual blood, crops do not put forth shoots, wine turns sour, grasses die, trees lose their fruit, iron is corrupted by rust, copper blackens, if dogs eat it they become rabid. Asphalt glue, which cannot be melted by fire or dissolved by water, when it is tainted by this blood, disintegrates by itself.'

The symptoms of menopause – episodes of heat, emotional mood swings, depression, sexual dysfunction and even osteoporotic fractures have been described in early Egyptian, Greek, Persian, Roman, Arabic, Chinese and Indian texts.[2] However, it is difficult to determine whether these symptoms were recorded as a sequel to, or consistently associated with, absence of the menstrual bleed. Both the ancient Hippocratic and Aristotle schools of health and hygiene in Greece postulated that as a woman aged, she no longer produced the nourishment necessary to form menstrual blood.

Women's bodies were deemed to be cold and wet and those of men to be warm and dry. It was thought that a man sweats to rid himself of his impurities whereas a woman bleeds. The absence of blood at the menopause was regarded as a 'negative' as the impurities and toxins were thought to be retained within the body and to wreak havoc in it. It was the accepted belief in those early days that, because of lack of nourishment, women became drier and colder but historical records do not record whether flushes and sweats were associated with the time when a woman ceased to menstruate.

In 1597, when Sir William Monson's wife consulted Simon Forman '*she had not had her course and the menstrual blood runneth to her head*', he recorded, and she was '*much subject to melancholy and full of fancies*'.[3]

One of the first gynaecological handbooks, written by a woman, described the menopause thus '*because there are many women who numerous diverse illnesses, some of them almost fatal*'. It was thought that women had less heat in their bodies than men, and had more moisture because their lack of heat would not dry their moisture and their humours. The menstrual bleeding was thought to make their bodies clean and whole. When they ceased menstruating at the time of their menopause, the toxic humours were retained, causing psychological and other maladies.[4]

There in a short sentence, ladies, is an old slant on the reason for your 'moments'!

It appears that the symptoms currently acknowledged as being present in a woman experiencing the menopause were recorded as occurring in older women, but the account by early Greek scholars, of coldness and dryness in older women, is in contrast to the modern portrayal of the post-menopause phase as being associated with flushes, sweats, insomnia and emotional instability.[5] Perhaps the description of coldness reflected the strained interpersonal relationships which frequently develop between older couples, whether occurring 2500 years ago or in the present era, while the dryness may refer to the loss of skin collagen or to the thin, dry, inelastic vaginal epithelium (the lining of the vagina). During the 2000 to 3000 years extending from recorded historical times to the 20th century, a variety of therapy programs were prescribed to treat some of the individual symptoms which a woman had been experiencing, all with varying degrees of success.

Chamomile, vitex (chaste tree), sage leaf, panax ginseng, licorice, tribulus, motherwort, dandelion and hypericum perforatum (St John's Wort) were just some of the plants used extensively by Chinese and Indian herbalists in pre-Christian times while others mixed various combinations of herbs, mushrooms and plant roots to treat the 'instability' experienced by an older woman. The first pharmacopaea, (the Shennong Bencao Jing) was written during the Han Dynasty (about 200 years BC) and described a variety of plant and fungal extracts to maintain and improve the body equilibrium. Lingzhi was the fungus of choice for treating most women with what could be considered menopausal symptoms. Even today, extracts of these plants and fungi are often the preferred treatment regimens by a very large number of women, not only in Asian countries but also in Western society.

Other cultures (including American Indians who used the extract of black cohosh to reduce fever, sweats and flushes) used a variety of herbs and plant extracts to relieve symptoms of menopause and, in recent times, extracts of these plants have been studied in order to determine if any contain chemicals that can be applied in 'modern' medicine.

Dong Quai, bupleurum, atractylodes, ginger and salvia roots have all been used in various combinations to produce Chinese herbal medicines to treat menopause symptoms but no single substance has been identified as having a major and sustained influence on reducing the distressing symptoms of estrogen deficiency.

These plant and herbal preparations were the only medications available for symptoms peculiar to older women during this time in history, but unfortunately they do not relieve the complaints of the vast majority of contemporary women who continue to experience the severe or disabling results of hormone deficiency. It is only in the last 150 years that a concerted effort has been made to understand the menopause and to determine the cause so that a program of treatment which would cure the symptoms could be developed.

In the early 19th century, French physicians, who first observed a connection between the development of flushes and the menopause, clinically identified an association between cessation of menstrual periods and the onset of menopausal symptoms.

A history of management of the menopause

The young English physician John Tilt wrote the first of his articles on the health of women after he returned from Paris in 1839.[6] He had trained for a time in Paris and was one of the first to recognise that the ovary was responsible for a number of reproductive and feminine functions in a woman – menstruation, pregnancy and menopause, and he also believed that any 'madness' that afflicted women during the peri-menopause, was caused by the ovaries. He promoted the hypothesis in the 1840s that most disabilities suffered by women were ovarian in origin and could be cured by surgical removal of the ovaries, an operation in which he and other surgeons became adept. This surgery, which had a high death rate, showed little evidence of improved behaviour, no relief of symptoms, and created a marked loss of a woman's sexual desire.[7]

Fortunately, by 1880, the operation had been totally abandoned as a treatment of hysteria and female psychiatric disorders.

In spite of evidence that these bizarre interventions were cruel and unnecessary, a woman of the 19th century, entering her menopause, continued to be treated in a shameful way by doctors and it was not until social changes and feminine pressure encouraged doctors to investigate and view the menopause as a life event requiring 'treatment' that advances and understanding occurred.

The 20th century introduced the beginning of a greater understanding about hormones and their importance in maintaining the health of the individual, with the initial major breakthroughs in endocrinology taking place in the understanding and treatment of diabetes, of thyroid function and also of the menopause.

Sex and its influence on the understanding of the menopause

For hundreds of years, when a woman became menopausal and her vagina became dry or tight, lacking the normal elasticity necessary for sexual intercourse, when she became osteoporotic or when she developed mental or psychological dysfunction, it became acceptable in some societies for a married man to take a younger mistress in order to satisfy his sexual desires and inclination. During the 16th, 17th and 18th centuries unconstrained sexual activity between consenting adults was accepted as normal; to be enjoyed by both men and women with plays and books being written regarding the pleasure to be obtained by such indulgence both within and outside marriage. It was not until the Victorian era that such 'licentious' attitudes began to change and extra-marital relationships were frowned upon. Even within marriage, sexual enjoyment was regarded as a sign of wanton behaviour.

By the beginning of the 19th century it was recognised that some of the symptoms and abnormal behaviours exhibited by women were associated with ovarian dysfunction. The severity, and censorious attitude of Victorian prudery, became pre-eminent, particularly regarding sexual freedom for women, and a number of books were written by learned physicians extolling the virtue of sexual intercourse – but only for procreation within a marriage – not for a woman's pleasure! Sexual enjoyment or promiscuity, particularly by a post-menopausal woman, was regarded as being un-Godly and required both surgical and spiritual intervention. The promiscuous behaviour of some women was regarded as 'an ominous sign of national decay'.

It was not until the later stages of the 19th century that women began once more to express their desire to contribute to, and enjoy, a different role in society. Some women even declared their desire to participate in sexual activity purely for pleasure. But because of changes in their vagina this became impossible for a large number of them who, having run out of eggs in their ovaries, were lacking estrogen and had entered their menopause.

Women demanded some medical therapy to prevent hot flushes and also to improve the dry, inelastic lining of their vagina. Sexual intercourse had become a painful and distressing event and this not only resulted in loss of libido but also accentuated marital conflict and their partner's infidelity. The need to improve the quality of life and the sexual anatomy of post-menopausal women had become not only a medical issue but a social issue as well.

Many different therapies and devices were developed in an attempt to maintain the sexual feminine allure of a peri-menopausal woman. These ranged from vaginal lubricants to magic potions, herbs and spices and even the use of mechanical devices. It was not until the 1930s that estrogens were introduced with the express purpose of improving the quality of life for a woman whose future was being seriously disrupted by menopausal symptoms.

While knowledge about the hormonal changes involved in the menopause has increased exponentially over the past 100 years, there are still many myths, lies, distortions, doubts, and scepticisms surrounding it, resulting in misunderstanding of the menopause, the scientific evidence of the value of estrogen and of the various alternative treatment options.

Over the last 100 years, the connection between ovarian failure and a variety of clinical symptoms and signs has been identified and the cause is much clearer. As a result, the role of estrogen in maintaining a woman's health has become evident and most modern treatments are now based on replacing this hormone. More recently, however, adverse reports suggesting that estrogen therapy caused breast cancer have achieved prominence, and as a result a 'climate of fear' has developed regarding the use of hormone therapy.

A woman usually decides to begin estrogen-based hormone therapy because she is experiencing hot flushes, sweats, insomnia or marked vaginal discomfort as she enters the menopause. For over 70 years, women have been happy to obtain relief from these distressing post-menopausal symptoms through use of estrogen therapy. As a bonus, positive reports from multiple clinical research and observational studies have also reported a reduced risk of osteoporotic fractures, a reduction in cardiovascular disease and a reduced incidence of dementia when using Hormone Replacement Therapy (HRT).

The euphoria surrounding various hormone therapy treatments was interrupted by the publication of the Women's Health Initiative report in 2002. Since 2002, use of hormone therapy has often been rejected by women and many have made a conscious decision to avoid using any hormone therapy because of the fear that hormones will cause some adverse effect such as breast cancer. However, it is worth reviewing the historical facts in order to fully appreciate the role that estrogen plays in the health of a woman.

Because of the need to treat the distressing symptoms of menopause and to avoid the perceived risk of breast cancer, various fungal, herbal and other plant extracts have been extensively promoted and proclaimed as being viable alternative therapies. Some of the claims have been based on the knowledge that the plants contain large amounts of phyto-estrogens which are frequently recommended as having a beneficial effect on symptoms while others have relied on the fact that some plant extracts have been used in traditional medicine for generations. For many individuals suffering severe symptoms, the success of these plant extracts has been less than expected or as advertised.

By the beginning of the 21st century, clinical trials were being conducted to determine the efficacy of these plant-derived therapies. One randomised, placebo-controlled trial comparing the effectiveness of black cohosh, red clover extract, estradiol and a placebo, resulted in the remission of flushes and sweats after one year for each of these treatments, but red clover extract failed to be as effective as the placebo, and the black cohosh was even less effective.[8]

Placebo is a medical term for a medicine that performs no physiological function but may benefit the patient psychologically. It is taken from the Latin *'I shall please'* that has been adapted as more to please than to benefit the patient. Placebos were widespread in medicine until the 20th century and they were sometimes endorsed as 'necessary deceptions' because in the words of Ambroise Pare (1510–1590) the duty of physicians is 'to cure occasionally, relieve often, console always'.

In spite of thousands of years of the use of 'natural' products, and an accumulated experience regarding their application, the persistence of the disabling effects of estrogen deficiency has resulted in a large proportion of women requesting a more active and reliable therapy program to overcome the distressing symptoms of menopause.

The development of effective hormone therapy

When research identified the ovary as the body's source of the hormones that are needed to induce sexual changes in a woman, there was a huge interest in developing preparations of these hormones so that youthful sexual responses in a woman could be maintained after her ovaries no longer produced them.

From the late 19th century doctors had been extracting small quantities of hormones from animal ovaries and had injected these extracts into women, but the limited ability to obtain sufficient amounts of these hormones and the poor results which followed soon led to a decline in the use of this method of hormone replacement. However, as scientists continued to identify the complex molecular structure of hormones produced by the ovary and the testicle, it became a feasible idea that a suitable estrogen would soon be synthesised to replace natural estrogen.

In the beginning of the quest to obtain the 'right' ovarian hormone, it was believed that only estrone was produced, but later it was discovered that the ovary produced estradiol as the primary estrogen, and that this hormone was later metabolised to estrone by enzymes throughout other parts of the body. Progesterone and testosterone were not considered to be essential ovarian hormones until some years after the discovery of estrone and estradiol.

Estrogen

Estrogen is the name given to a group of *natural* hormones that include estradiol, estrone and estriol. Estradiol is the primary estrogen produced by the ovary. It is the most potent estrogen and is the estrogen most used in HRT. Estradiol is reduced by enzymes in the body to the weaker estrogen *estrone* and then to the even weaker estrogen *estriol.*

Synthesised ethinyl estradiol was the estrogen used initially but this has since been superseded in post-menopausal therapy regimens by bio-identical estradiol.

A chemical with estrogenic properties, Bisphenol-A (BPA), was invented in 1891. It is an interesting solid plastic that is now used worldwide in a huge range of domestic and commercial products. It was recognised that Bisphenol-A had estrogenic properties when administered to laboratory animals but it was never used in a form suitable for women to relieve their symptoms of the menopause. Recently there has been increasing interest in the possibility that molecules of BPA may leach out of plastic bottles and other household goods to induce a variety of adverse effects, including breast cancer and also genetic mutations in infants using feeding bottles made with BPA. By the 1930s, BPA was discarded as a possible model of an estrogen as scientists explored other chemicals that were being designed and could be used in order to produce a beneficial effect in women.

Professor Dodds in the United Kingdom invented diethylstilboestrol (DES) in 1936, followed soon after by German scientists who, in 1938, invented the synthesised estrogen, *ethinyl estradiol.* Over the following 20 years both these estrogenic products were used to treat a variety of diseases and hormone-related problems, including threatened abortion, premature labour, breast cancer and osteoporosis. Within two decades of its discovery and clinical development, the synthesised hormone, ethinyl estradiol, began to be used as the estrogen of choice in the majority of oral contraceptive pills. The development of the contraceptive pill is an important step to the development of HRT for the treatment of the symptoms of the menopause. During the early years of estrogen therapy, ethinyl estradiol was also promoted in Europe as being an effective therapeutic agent for treatment of menopause symptoms, but by the late 1960s it was superseded by bio-identical estradiol as the estrogen of choice in hormone programs.

In the late 1930s, it was recognised that pregnant mares produced copious amounts of equine estrogens, of which the major portion was the biologically inert estrone sulphate. The Ayerst/Wyeth Pharmaceutical Company extracted the conglomerate of equine estrogens from pregnant mares' urine, and by 1942, it was marketing the complex of estrogens as Premarin. By removing the sulphate molecule, the estrone sulphate in Premarin is readily converted, by sulphatase enzymes in fat and liver cells of women, into the biologically active compounds, estrone and estradiol. The highly potent estradiol is normally rapidly metabolised by dehydrogenase enzymes in the human female to estrone and ultimately to the very weak estriol before it is excreted.

Because these metabolic changes to Premarin result in a number of estrogens identical to human estrogens, it is often regarded as being a 'natural' hormone. During the 60 years following its introduction, Premarin became the premier estrogenic hormone sold in the United States, and the majority of menopause studies in North America used Premarin as the estrogen of choice in HRT-related research.

Bio-identical hormones

Bio-identical hormones have been produced in laboratories since the late 1940s by a process involving enzymatic conversion of a substrate. (A substrate is any substance, which, by itself has no major identified action but which can be converted by an enzyme to produce an active compound). Because the substrate (diosgenin) is usually obtained from plants such as Mexican wild yam or from soy seed it has been claimed by proponents of alternative therapy programs that such plant-derived bio-identical hormones are more 'natural' than hormones used in regular commercial therapy. However, the hormones used by alternative therapists and by regular pharmaceutical companies are usually produced by the same chemical process, and may even be obtained from the same laboratory. The estradiol that is produced for both alternative and for regular commercial therapies has the same molecular structure

Enzymes are the protein 'workforce' of cells. Enzymes are specific proteins that catalyse (assist) a specific activity in a cell in order to achieve a metabolic function or outcome. Most enzyme-initiated activity is very rapid, taking seconds to start a chemical reaction. Bio-identical estradiol, synthesised in a laboratory, has been used in most commercial pharmaceutical preparations of hormone therapy for over 50 years. However, because oral estradiol is rapidly metabolised, or broken down within minutes, by enzymes in the gut and liver to the less active molecule estrone, scientists have developed a method to block the enzyme responsible for degrading the estradiol by temporarily attaching a side-chain molecule to the estradiol (conjugation) to slow the metabolic breakdown process. This allows for the administration of a lower dose of a hormone that is longer lasting (for between ten and sixteen hours) and is more effective, providing a safer level of estradiol to be taken by mouth.

Some doctors and promoters of alternative therapies have suggested that there is a difference between the estradiol produced by pharmaceutical companies for use in regular HRT therapy, and the estradiol used in alternative programs for transdermal (through the skin) or transbuccal (through the mucous membrane of the mouth) delivery but in fact, the molecules are identical and estradiol available in both regular and alternative HRT may even be produced in the same laboratory.

In 1965, Professor Diczfalusy[9] in Sweden discovered Estetrol, a fetal oestrogen that is produced only in the liver of a fetus (a baby still in the womb). It is a potent estrogen that, in a woman, has the ability to protect the bone from osteoporosis as well as inhibiting symptoms of the menopause. In research using animals, Estetrol also appeared to be capable of protecting against breast cancer. Estetrol may prove to be the most effective estrogen for the treatment of a post-menopausal woman, but this requires further research to determine its full potential.

Progesterone/Progestogens

Progesterone is one of the natural hormones produced by the ovary in the second half of a menstrual cycle, and also produced at a high level by the placenta during pregnancy. Oral progesterone is very rapidly metabolised by enzymes, particularly in the gut and liver, to substances that have no protective effect on women. Therefore the development of stable chemicals with a progesterone-like action became a necessity to enable doctors to safely treat a post-menopausal woman with estrogen.

Progestogen is the name applied to any chemical, which induces a progesterone-like effect on the endometrium of the uterus. In the United States, the term 'progestin' is used instead of 'progestogen' but the two terms are synonymous and refer to the same family of synthesised chemicals.

All steroid hormones including estradiol, progesterone and testosterone are derived from the cholesterol molecule and although they induce very different responses within cells, they differ from each other by only a few molecules at particular sites. The molecular changes that make any one of the steroid sex hormones differ one from the other, are carried out by specific enzymes found in granulosa cells that surround an egg. When a woman runs out of eggs and granulosa cells no longer develop, no more enzymes are available and therefore no further sex hormones are produced by the ovary. She has reached her menopause!

In 1937, a biochemical scientist, Russell Marker[10], described the chemical process that allowed him to synthesise and manufacture large quantities of bio-identical progesterone from a chemical precursor called diosgenin. Diosgenin is found in many plants, but Marker required a readily available and plentiful source of the substrate. He abandoned his university position and, on a field trip to Mexico he found the Mexican wild yam that contains large amounts of diosgenin. Using enzymes, he was able to convert diosgenin into bio-identical progesterone. The transformation of diosgenin substrate from plants into progesterone that is bio-identical to human progesterone then allowed clinicians to have access to a plentiful supply of relatively cheap bio-identical progesterone for clinical use.

However, the rapid breakdown of progesterone by enzymes in the gut and liver resulted in this bio-identical progesterone being unacceptable to prescribing doctors because long-lasting and reliable suppression of growth of the endometrium lining the uterus could not be achieved.

Obtaining a prolonged and high level of progesterone is also important to suppress the hypothalamic/pituitary centre of the brain that controls ovarian function. This requirement was vitally important when considering a hormone for use in developing oral contraceptives. Because bio-identical progesterone is broken down so rapidly it was unsuitable to achieve a reliable level of hormone suppression over a longer period of time. For this reason, stable synthesised steroid molecules that had an action similar to the action of progesterone were developed. These hormones are known as 'synthetic' progestogens/progestins in order to differentiate them from the rapidly metabolised bio-identical progesterone. These synthesised steroids are used in all oral contraceptives as well as in the majority of commercially designed menopause therapy programs. They have been confirmed by numerous studies as having a protective effect on the endometrium as well as suppressing cell activity in the hypothalamic/ pituitary region of the brain.

Although the synthetic progestogens have been promoted as superior to bio-identical progesterone for endometrial protection, research has demonstrated that an oral capsule containing 200mg of micronised progesterone is also capable of inducing a secretory effect in the endometrium.

While oral micronised progesterone is capable of being absorbed and passing from the gut to the liver, where it can enter the circulation to protect the endometrium, there is clear evidence that transdermal progesterone (applied as a cream to the skin) has no such protective effect. In one study from the Sydney Menopause Centre in 2002[11], it was concluded that the use of the transdermal route to administer progesterone did not allow sufficient amounts of the hormone to enter the circulation to achieve a biological effect on lipid (blood fats) levels, bone mineral metabolic indicators, vaso-motor symptoms (flushes, sweats) or on mood.

Another study from the same Menopause Department using transdermal (skin application) progesterone cream failed to produce any effect on the endometrium, on bleeding pattern, or on the plasma or salivary levels of progesterone.[12] A similar study in the United Kingdom in 2009 during which progesterone cream was evaluated in 223 women over 24 weeks, failed to show any benefit for relief of menopausal symptoms.[13]

The development of oral contraception and HRT

From 1950 onwards, most research into the use of sex hormones revolved around the development of an oral contraceptive. In order to ensure a reliable level of estrogen and progestogen, the pioneers of oral contraception such as Professors Pincus, Rock, Rice-Wray and others chose the stable ethinyl estradiol (EE) as the estrogen and employed either medroxyprogesterone acetate (Provera) or norethisterone (norethindrone) acetate as the progestogen for the 'new' oral contraceptive pill formulations.

A number of articles have been published over the past 50 years extolling the virtues of oral contraceptives, with the most comprehensive long-term study of the use of oral contraceptives demonstrating that women, using a progestogen/progestin with ethinyl estradiol in various oral contraceptive preparations, have a significant beneficial long-term health outcome compared to women who never use oral contraceptives. The Royal College of General Practitioners Oral Contraceptive Study[14] was begun in 1968 and recruited 46,112 women who required contraception and who were then followed for 39 years. It was found that women who used oral contraceptives had a significantly lower rate of death from all causes than never users. Rates of death from all cancers (including bowel, uterus and ovary), circulatory diseases (heart attacks and hypertension) and other diseases were 12 per cent lower than among women who had never taken 'the pill'.

Although during the past 50 years millions of women have used oral contraceptives containing higher doses of much more potent synthetic estrogens and progestogens than is contained in HRT, there has never been the same orchestrated media outcry or public reaction against oral contraceptive hormones as has occurred for similar therapy programs which use a lower dose of bio-identical estradiol, with a synthetic progestogen, for post-menopausal women.

The development of Hormone Replacement Therapy

The difficulties associated with the development of HRT have been related to the way that hormones, particularly estrogen and progesterone are utilised and degraded in a woman's body. The ovary continuously releases estradiol in very small amounts. However, progesterone is released in relatively large amounts in the second half of the menstrual cycle from an active corpus luteum in the ovary. However when prescribed and given by mouth the breakdown of these two hormones in the gut and liver has resulted in the need to develop alternative ways of giving these hormones. The use of gels, patches and implants has provided an alternative method of having hormone therapy.

In the 1960s, when it was realised that the same hormones used for contraception could also be used to treat menopause symptoms, research was begun into the various combinations, routes of delivery, dosages and types of estrogens and progestogens currently available and which were considered suitable for a woman in her post-menopause years.

In Europe, ethinyl estradiol, a synthesised stable estrogen, was the most common estrogen used, while in the United States, Premarin extracted from the urine of pregnant mares, was used as the basis of most hormone replacement therapies.

When developing therapies to treat menopausal symptoms, the oral use of bio-identical progesterone was not initially considered because of its inadequate action on the endometrium. Also taken into consideration were the results of prior research on oral contraceptives. The availability of the more stable and cheaper synthesised progestogens resulted in a more reliable product.

By the late 1960s, hormone therapy was widely accepted and women were told that their menopause problems could be solved. Dr Robert A. Wilson[15] published his book *Feminine Forever* and women of the world embraced the use of HRT.

During the 50 years following publication of Wilson's book, research into the benefits of HRT confirmed that estrogen therapy resulted in remission of flushes and sweats as well as inducing a dramatic benefit to the dry, inelastic vaginal epithelium (lining of the vagina).

Substantial clinical evidence from studies designed to observe the effect of estrogen on the health of post-menopausal women had begun to accumulate, suggesting that estrogen, begun at the time of the menopause, reduced the risk of osteoporosis and fractures in a woman,[16] reduced the incidence of atherosclerosis and heart attacks,[17] reduced the incidence of dementia[18] and extended the life of a post-menopausal woman.[19]

Pharmaceutical companies competed to produce better and more varied therapies but the plethora of treatment options was dramatically interrupted in 2002 following the publication of the Women's Health Initiative (WHI) Study with the associated hysteria and fear engendered by claims that hormones caused breast cancer.

During the years that have elapsed since estrogen was introduced in the 1930s, research in clinical departments in many countries around the world was accumulating to suggest that a woman who began using hormone therapy to alleviate the distressing symptoms of flushes, sweats, insomnia, mood swings or a dry uncomfortable vagina, also had a reduced risk of heart attacks and premature death.

By the mid 1980s these observational studies had provided such compelling evidence that estrogens, begun at the time a woman passed the menopause, prevented cardiovascular damage, physicians contended that if estrogen was capable of preventing heart attacks, it might also be of benefit to women who already had suffered damage to their coronary vessels.

To explore the possibility that estrogen might be able to reverse the damaging effect of atherosclerosis, a major prospective placebo-controlled study was initiated (the famous Hormone and Estrogen/Progestin Replacement (HERS) study). Physicians recruited 2763 women who had either suffered a coronary occlusion or had had bypass surgery or coronary artery stents.[20] The average age of these women was 67 years (15–20 years after passing their menopause) and they had an average body mass index (BMI) of 29 (in the overweight category). Unfortunately, the use of estrogen (Premarin) was not able to initially improve the outcome – in fact, in the first year there was an increased risk of thrombosis and death among the women using the hormone therapy. Following publication of the HERS results in 1998 it was advised that post-menopausal women with known cardiovascular damage should not be prescribed oral estrogen therapy.

When women reach the menopause, the majority of them are found to have an excellent cardiovascular system. However, within a decade after their menopause, and without the protection of estrogen, many of them will develop some arterial damage with deposits of cholesterol in the arteries, and are at risk of atherosclerosis (hardening of the arteries) and thrombosis. Unfortunately by the time the HERS paper had been published the National Institute of Health had already recruited 161,700 women of whom two-thirds were over the age of 60 years for the huge Women's Health Initiative Study. A large number of the women recruited to the WHI Study were similar in demographic background to the women in the HERS Study – they were already post-menopausal, 75 per cent had not had estrogen for fifteen to twenty years and two-thirds were overweight.

What the HERS Study showed was that the use of oral estrogen was contraindicated in older women who already had damaged arteries – the WHI Study results published four years later also confirmed that many women beginning *oral* HRT ten to 30 years after their menopause had double the risk of premature death than women who had not begun any therapy at the time of their menopause.

The increased risk of thrombosis and heart attacks in both the HERS and WHI Study was thought to be related to three major problems:

1. The late age when estrogen was initiated.
2. The use of *oral* estrogen therapy. (The liver is the primary source of the various proteins that cause blood to clot. Estrogen absorbed from the gut and passing directly to the liver stimulates the liver to increase the production of these clotting factors.)
3. The underlying physical disadvantages of overweight, hypertensive, diabetic women who smoked and who had elevated cholesterol levels.

If hormone therapy is required for women with risk of cardiovascular disease, then transdermal or transbuccal therapy is thought to be the best way of providing estradiol.

Summary

For over 2000 years, menstruation and menopause have been clouded in mystery. The legends conceived by ancient philosophers were their attempts to explain events that they could not understand.

To alleviate symptoms of the menopause, women resorted to the use of folk medicine and herbal concoctions suggested by wise women of the village or compounded by apothecaries.

Women of the 19th century were treated during the menopause with cruel and unnecessary and bizarre interventions including the removal of their ovaries in order to cure them of their 'hysteria'. Towards the end of the Victorian era, women became emancipated and wanted sexual enjoyment. They requested therapies to alleviate their symptoms of menopause and to improve their sex life.

During the 20th century with the advancement of endocrinology, the mysteries and beliefs of menstruation and the menopause began to be more fully understood, with the development of the oral contraceptive 'pill' and more sophisticated therapies for the relief of symptoms of the menopause.

In the last 80 years, many new scientific and medical discoveries have helped to dispel the myths surrounding the mystery of a woman's body. These discoveries have also enabled progress in the development of suitable hormone therapies, particularly estrogen and progesterone.

These developments also provide a woman with options in hormone therapies that can alleviate many of the symptoms of the menopause, as well as reduce the impact of diseases that, after her menopause, can reduce a woman's quality of life and life expectancy.

Unfortunately, the negative publicity at the beginning of the 21st century regarding the misinterpretation of the Women's Health Initiative report resulted in a prejudicial impression regarding the therapy options available to the health of post-menopausal women.

CHAPTER 2

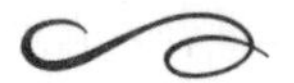

The anatomy and physiology of the menopause

A single moment of understanding can flood a whole life with meaning.

—Anonymous

Menopause

The menopause is just one day in a woman's life. It is the last day she has a menstrual bleed. It usually occurs between the age of 45 and 55 years and is caused by her ovaries running out of eggs and their consequent failure to produce a woman's sex hormones, particularly estrogen, progesterone and testosterone.

The word *menopause*, coined in 1832 from the Greek root *men-* (month) and word *pausis* (cessation), literally means 'the end of monthly cycles'. The word was created to describe this change in human females, when the end of fertility is traditionally indicated by the *permanent* ending of monthly bleeding.

The menopause is usually associated with the onset of uncomfortable flushes (flashes) or episodes of heat that suffuse the body and face of a woman, and are caused by a sudden surge of blood in the capillaries supplying the skin of the face, neck and body. During these episodes, or vaso-motor symptoms, the skin temperature may rise by 0.5 to 2.5 degrees celsius and can be associated with sweating, dizziness and palpitations. These episodes of flushes, usually last for 1 to 5 minutes and are more frequent at night, often waking her and resulting in insomnia and tiredness, loss of energy and, for some women, severe emotional and psychological disturbance. Some women have a flush every 20 to 30 minutes while others have only an occasional mild flush once in a day. While about

20 per cent of women never experience flushes or sweats, among the 80 per cent who do suffer from symptoms, about half find they are not too bothersome or that they gradually diminish within five years. But for at least 40 per cent, these distressing vaso-motor symptoms continue to disturb a woman for the remainder of her life. It is important to realise that the presence or absence of hot flushes and sweats is not an indication of other changes in a woman's body. Some women boast that they 'sailed' through the menopause with no problems, only to suffer an osteoporotic fracture when they were in their sixties or to develop dementia when in their seventies.

The difficulty of terminology of 'the menopause' is that there are actually three stages of it but very little understanding of them. These three stages are: the peri-menopause which includes the menopause transition as well as the year after the final menstrual bleed; the menopause which is a point in time; and the post-menopause which lasts for the rest of a woman's life. Possibly the most bewildering of these three stages is the first stage: the years of the peri-menopause.

Peri-menopause

The peri-menopause starts when the ovaries begin to run out of eggs and is complete 12 months after the last menstrual period has occurred. In the few years before complete cessation of menstrual periods, the number of eggs left in the ovaries is usually insufficient to continue the normal ovulation process, pregnancy is generally no longer possible and the amount of estrogen and progesterone being secreted is low or absent, resulting in very irregular 'periods'. The peri-menopause is often associated with irregular, heavy bleeding and marked mood changes, with intermittent episodes of hot flushes, sweats, insomnia and loss of libido. It has been determined that the *average* age for an Australian woman to begin her peri-menopause is about 46 years. The menopause has, over recorded history, presented with many different symptoms and physical changes for different women, with some having no symptoms through the 'change' while others experience debilitating and distressing ones. This is when many women seek medical help, but their problems are often not recognised as being related to the peri-menopause. The term *menopausal transition* describes the final years of the peri-menopause leading up to the final menstrual period.[21] The menopause transition is a phase of the peri-menopause when symptoms are more intense.

The ovaries begin to decline after a woman reaches the age of about 35 years. This gradual decline begins to gain momentum any time after she is about 40 years, and when her eggs and their follicles decline in number the ovaries release less estrogen. It is the fall in the level of estrogen that initiates the symptoms of the peri-menopause and it is particularly distressing for a woman who has dramatic peaks and lows within her menstrual cycle. This lability or period of unstable hormone release is also the cause of the symptoms of premenstrual tension (PMT).

Blood levels of anti-Mullerian hormone (AMH), estradiol and the follicle stimulating hormone (FSH) are tests that can help determine when a woman is in the peri-menopause.

There are over 40 symptoms that may be associated with the peri-menopause. They begin to mark a physiological change in a woman's body and every woman's response to this change may be different. Many believe that the typical woman in 'menopause' experiences hot flushes, that she gains weight and has mood swings, but it is known that up to 20 per cent of women have no symptoms at all. Other women experience the symptoms of the peri-menopause in varying degrees. Even though her ovaries are failing and hormone production fluctuates widely, it is still possible for a woman to conceive naturally in the peri-menopause.

A woman's body adapts to changing hormone levels throughout her lifetime, but when changes are most dramatic such as during pregnancy or in the peri-menopause, she may need therapeutic support to maintain her psychological as well as her physiological equilibrium. In the peri-menopause, symptoms and signs become manifest when a woman's sex hormone levels fluctuate widely or too rapidly. The level of estrogen, progesterone, testosterone, follicle-stimulating hormone (FSH) and luteinising hormone (LH) fluctuate and may change from very little detected in the circulation to huge levels in the space of a few days. These widely variable hormone levels during the peri-menopause may induce abrupt and intermittent mood swings, temperamental outbursts and episodes of abnormal behaviour.

When a woman is under pressure because of factors such as chronic stress, inadequate sleep, a poor diet, too little exercise and also environmental influences, it is very difficult for her to cope with the fluctuations of her hormone levels. This is when things begin to 'fall apart' and she experiences symptoms and signs of the peri-menopause to a greater degree. Many women are surprised by the wide range of symptoms associated with the peri-menopause and also that these symptoms can appear long before, or in addition to, the classic sign of the peri-menopause – heavy or irregular periods. The most common of these early symptoms include irritability, depressed mood, weight gain, fuzzy thinking, anxiety and headaches.

Possibly the most distressing of these symptoms are mood swings, irritability and anxiety because they have a ripple effect on a woman's daily life. A woman's relationships, both personal and in the workplace, become strained and her family can be severely affected by her tiredness and her emotional outbursts. These events are similar to those experienced in pre-menstrual tension and it is a clinical observation that a woman who already has pre-menstrual tension (PMT) may be more predisposed to hormonal and neurotransmitter imbalance in the peri-menopause. These emotional changes appear to be related to the erratic hormonal fluctuations that occur in the days before menstruation as well as in the time of her menopause transition. The good news is that when the menopause has passed and the symptoms of hormone fluctuations have disappeared, the post-menopause years proceed more calmly.

Peri-menopause is the interval in which a woman's body makes a natural shift from fairly regular cycles of ovulation and menstruation toward permanent infertility or menopause. This shift is generally first noticed when a woman is in her mid forties but the signs might be noticed in her thirties. Her periods can become irregular – longer or shorter, heavier or lighter and her usual cycle may become less reliable. Not only does she have menstrual irregularity, but also other more subtle changes can begin to disrupt her life.

Hot flushes and night sweats can disturb her sleep; she may notice changes in bladder function; she may experience sexual discomfort because her estrogen levels are no longer sufficient to maintain her vaginal tissues. This also leaves her more vulnerable to urinary and vaginal infections. Her libido also lessens because her falling levels of estrogen and testosterone affect the areas of her brain that 'turn her on'. Memory is part of an individual, but when her brain no longer receives its fair share of estrogen a woman will notice that she forgets many things – appointments, invitations, facts and figures. Sometimes forgetting her own telephone number can be distressing for her as well as overlooking the commitments that she has made to her children.

As a woman's estrogen level falls, her harmful cholesterol (LDL) level may rise. This is one of the 'silent' signs of peri-menopause and can be particularly harmful for her in her post-menopause years. The same concern exists for the health of her bones. For these reasons it is advisable for a woman of 50 years to have annual medical and gynaecological checks. Any symptom of the peri-menopause can be helped with the advice of her medical practitioner and in some cases medication can be used. The use of a low dose contraceptive pill is a suitable option to control hormone dysfunction as well as preventing an unwanted pregnancy.

Penelope's story

Menopause was the worst possible time in my life. From the age of 50 to 52 it was sheer hell. Yes, I had the obvious symptoms - itchy skin, hot flushes, trouble sleeping, no interest in sex, but the worst thing was the incredible mood swings.

My poor husband, if ever he had reason to leave, it was during this time. However, he stood by me and tried to help, but I think at times, my behaviour was simply too bewildering for him as a man. I would be irrational, fly off the handle for no reason, and be totally unreasonable. Nobody in my family knew when they came home how they would find me ... moody, cranky ... just plain awful.

My garden became my solace.

I cried a great deal, morning, noon and night, for no reason. Without realising it I slid into a deep depression. I was on a fast downwards spiral. My bad behaviour had come to the notice of a friend and he called me and verbally stripped me of any dignity I may have still possessed. I was left shaking, bewildered and confused.

The truth always hurts and I quickly slid even deeper into depression and my denial of it. It was the only time in my life that I had contemplated suicide. The feelings of guilt and shame were unbearable, particularly as I began to feel that I had failed not only as a wife and mother but also as a friend.

During this time I knew that I should never have been driving. Even though I was usually a good driver, my concentration had gone and my reflexes were very poor.

Fortunately for me, a much loved girlfriend from interstate who had been through a breakdown some years beforehand, recognised my symptoms, arrived on my doorstep saying something like 'you can't go on like this, I have come to help you through this'. She took me to a doctor whom she felt could help me. This wonderful lady doctor took me under her wing, started me on HRT and counselled me for about six months. Thank God for HRT! Almost from the time I commenced it I had an amazing reversal of behaviour and remained on HRT for ten years.

Post-menopause

In Australia, between 3–4 million women in the population are now post-menopausal. Every year between 110,000–150,000 women pass from their peri-menopause into their post-menopause.

The post-menopause begins when a woman who has been in the peri-menopause has had no menstrual bleeding for twelve months or more. The post-menopause lasts for the remainder of a woman's life and it is in this phase that many adverse changes may take place. For women who suffer flushes and sweats, insomnia and mood disturbance, the need for symptom relief and emotional stability is paramount. These are the women who attend their doctor for advice, counselling and appropriate therapy. It is at this critical time in her life that a woman requires her doctor to provide accurate and unbiased information about the menopause, in order to allow her to make decisions about her post-menopausal years.

Premature menopause

Approximately 1 per cent of women will spontaneously enter the menopause before they have reached the age of 40 years because they have run out of viable eggs, while about another 5 per cent will have their ovaries removed during a surgical procedure or permanently injured following chemotherapy or irradiation for the treatment of a malignancy. The sudden loss of hormones in younger women may produce a more disastrous set of symptoms and adverse events than is experienced by women who gradually pass into the menopause over the years of the menopause transition. Not only are flushes, sweats and psychological disturbances a major problem, but women who have a premature menopause are more likely to experience an increase in cardiovascular diseases such as heart attacks, stroke and hypertension, as well as osteoporotic fractures and dementia. It is imperative that younger women who experience premature menopause are given appropriate therapy when their hormone levels are catastrophically diminished.

Bridgette's story

From a very young age I had always had a strong desire to have babies. At the age of 22, I fell pregnant. Being pregnant was a wonderful experience and I felt an absolute happiness when my son was born naturally on my birthday. I finally understood what an amazing gift mothers are given.

When my son was about three, I experienced my first hot flush. The sensation of heat travelling up my body soon became quite a regular thing. The next incident was when I waited for my period. As I had always been regular since I was 13, when I had missed the next period I thought I was pregnant but my pregnancy test was negative. Still no period and the hot flushes were coming fast and furious.

It wasn't until I had a pap smear and a cervical test and I mentioned my absent periods to the specialist. She asked me if I'd had a hormone test – I hadn't. Waiting for the results, I received devastating and unexpected news – the hormone reading was 'post-menopausal'. At the age of 26, I had just lost all the babies I had wished for. I never realised that early menopause existed. I was hysterical and couldn't be consoled. Immediately, the specialist suggested hormone replacement therapy to ease my symptoms, informing me that I would be on these drugs for the rest of my life.

I did try to go down the alternative therapies track with no success or proper support. The HRT was a godsend and my symptoms lessened, making me feel that my body was not quite so unpredictable.

Despite my early onset menopause, my partner and I started an assisted fertility program (Gamete Intro Fertilisation), which we attempted three times. This was unsuccessful so we were referred to another clinic for ovum donation. The stress on our relationship took its toll. At 30, I was a single mother, I had lost my house and any security I had. The ripple effect from my early menopause diagnosis impacted on so many areas of my life – it was so unlike anything I had imagined for my future, which was simply to be surrounded by my children.

I am now 40 and have come to a point in my life, even though the journey has been hard on me emotionally and physically, where I feel fortunate to have a child of my own.

For some women, the menopause is merely a minor change that they liken to walking through a doorway from one room to another – just requiring a modest alteration to their environment and way of life. However, for other women, it involves entering a long tunnel of despair where the future without treatment appears likely to be a miserable time.

Some critics of those providing treatment or offering therapy have claimed that the menopause is a disease invented by the pharmaceutical industry for financial gain, while others blame the medical profession for 'medicallising' a natural biological event. Yet, at the other extreme, women who are experiencing the adverse effects of the menopause have admonished many doctors for not recognising, or adequately treating, the physical, emotional and psychological symptoms associated with hormone deficiency.

The endocrine system

The medical discipline of endocrinology is the study of normal, as well as the management of abnormal hormone production. Gynaecological endocrinology is the study of hormones produced by, or which influence, ovarian function.

No normal cell in the body will perform any function or task unless it is given a message to do so. While certain messages, such as muscular movements are delivered rapidly by nerve impulses, the normal equilibrium and homeostasis of the body is carried out by steroid and protein messengers that circulate in the blood or pass directly from one cell to another. These messengers are called hormones.

Hormones are secreted into the blood from glands such as the pituitary, the thyroid, the thymus, the pancreas, the ovaries, the testicles, and many other endocrine cells such as in the stomach, the placenta, the kidneys and the heart. Almost all of them are controlled by the hypothalamus and the pituitary gland in the brain (see Appendix 8 for more information).

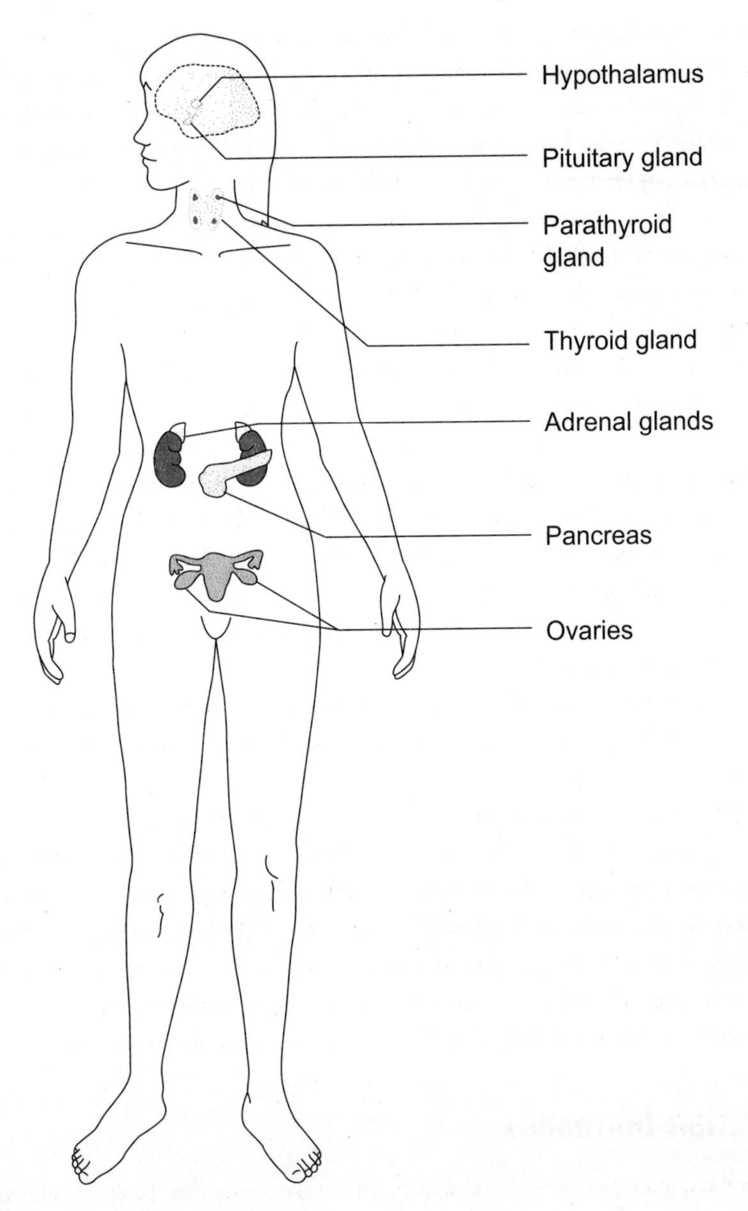

Figure 1. The endocrine system.

Hormones produced in any one of the many endocrine glands can enter cells as the blood circulates but a particular hormone will only induce an action if the cell has a receptor into which a hormone can fit and induce a response (very much like a key which may fit into a number of locks but will only turn the one which has been designed to match the key). Some hormones deliver the same message to every cell (insulin tells every cell to metabolise sugar) while other hormones may produce one response in one type of cell but a different response in another cell (testosterone may activate some cells in the skin to increase growth of hair but activates certain brain cells to perform an entirely different task). One of the estrogens, estradiol, may activate two entirely different receptors in the same cell and thus deliver two very different command messages to the same cell. So the response within a cell depends not only on the messenger (the hormone) but also on the protein receptor within the cell.

Hormones are the quiet guardians of our body. Endocrine glands and their hormones are responsible for maintaining the normal regularity and function of cells. There are multiple numbers of hormones and other controlling factors circulating in our body, and their main purpose is to maintain the internal environment of cells, and ultimately maintain the body in the stable and functional state of homeostasis. Hormones not only maintain normal cells, but they also determine how the body adapts to internal, as well as external environmental and other hostile conditions such as cancer, infections, cold, heat, thirst, starvation. Hormones instruct cells to respond to the altered conditions in a self-preserving fashion.

If one or more hormones are produced in excessive or insufficient amounts, the flow-on effects result in a marked disruption of the function of the human body.

The most common glands involved in a disruption within the endocrine system of a woman are the ovaries (menopause, infertility, PMS, abnormal menstrual pattern, etc.), the thyroid (myxoedema, hyperthyroidism), the pancreas (diabetes), the stomach (uncontrolled appetite – ghrelins, amylin), fat cells (obesity – amylin) and the adrenal and the pituitary glands. However, there are many other glands and hormones that contribute to the harmony of our body and disruption to one gland may adversely affect the actions of many others.

Ovarian hormones

The three main hormones produced by the ovary – estrogen, progesterone and testosterone are the ones that are described in this book.

Estrogen is the hormone that defines a woman and her femininity – it plays an essential role in the growth and development of her female characteristics and also in the reproductive process. 'Estrogen' is probably the most widely known of the ovarian hormones but in actual fact estrogen refers to a group of hormones which include estradiol, estrone and estriol.

ESTRADIOL
Estradiol is the most potent, naturally occurring estrogen in a woman.
Estradiol is the estrogen that is used in hormone therapy.

To understand the menopause and its significance for a woman, one must begin with an appreciation of what hormones are, what they do, what influence the 'sex' hormones have on the physiological function of a woman, and what happens to her when the ovaries cease producing the main sex hormones (estrogen, progesterone and testosterone).

Hormones are chemical messengers. This book is mainly concerned with the action of the ovarian hormones and the problems that develop in a woman who ceases producing sufficient estrogen, progesterone or testosterone from her ovaries. However, it must be remembered that many other hormones are also involved in maintaining the normal function and activity of cells, not only at the time of the menopause, but for life.

A good example of one of those hormones is insulin, which is secreted by the pancreas. Insulin circulates in the blood to tell every cell in our body to metabolise sugar for the energy that the cell needs to function properly. If the pancreas ceases to produce sufficient insulin, the cells fail to get the appropriate message, and although there is enough sugar in the circulation, metabolism of sugar within the cell stops, the level of blood sugar continues to rise and a diagnosis of diabetes is made. All that a diabetic person needs is to receive the right amount of insulin for the cells in order to begin to metabolise sugar again. The secret to successful management of a diabetic person is to administer the correct amount of insulin in the right way at the right time.

In a similar way, a post-menopausal woman whose ovaries have run out of eggs, stops producing the essential hormones (estradiol, progesterone, testosterone) normally secreted by the ovaries of young menstruating women. When the eggs in the ovary have been used up, the ovarian hormone levels fall dramatically. As a result, cells that have depended on these hormones fail to maintain their normal function.

Failure of the ovary to secrete its hormones is usually followed by physical changes and symptoms which may be so distressing for a woman that she will need these hormones, particularly estrogen in order for her cells to restore normal function, and to relieve her symptoms.

Anatomy of the reproductive organs of the pelvis

The uterus or womb is the organ in a woman where menstruation, implantation of a fertilised egg, the development of the baby and labour takes place. It is composed of smooth muscle cells that have the capacity to grow under the influence of the ovarian hormones. In a non-pregnant state the uterus is about 8–9 centimetres long but when a woman is pregnant, the uterus may grow to 40 centimetres in length. The lower section is about 2–3 centimetres long and has fibrous cells as well as muscle cells and this portion of the uterus is called the **cervix** (or neck of the uterus).

The inside of the uterus is lined with a special layer of glandular cells called the **endometrium**. Estradiol causes these endometrial cells to grow, in what is known as the **proliferative phase,** from a base thickness of 2–3mm to between 8 and 15mm within 10 to 15 days after the commencement of each menstrual cycle. When a woman ovulates and the ovary forms a corpus luteum producing progesterone, the secretory phase of the menstrual cycle is initiated, a process during which endometrial cells stop proliferating and fill up with nutritious secretions ready for a fertilised egg to implant. If there is no implantation of a fertilised egg, then the endometrial lining is shed off as a menstrual period.

The **vagina** is a flattened tube about 8–12 centimetres long that extends from the vulva to the cervix. The wall of the vagina is composed of four different layers – an inner layer of squamous cells similar to those of the skin, surrounded by a layer of collagen fibres that contains a rich supply of blood and lymph vessels. A third layer of smooth muscle fibres is arranged in a circular as well as a longitudinal direction and encircles these two layers. The fourth layer is composed of supportive tissue.

Normally, under the influence of estradiol, the vagina produces fluids composed of some secretions from the cervix but mostly some lymph fluid that oozes through the squamous layer from the copious supply of blood vessels and lymph vessels of the second layer. This vaginal fluid is mixed with dead cells shed from the vaginal wall and contains proteins, carbohydrates, amino acids, enzymes and aromatic compounds that is a source of nutrients for the normal organisms which grow readily in the moist warm environment. The dominant organism that inhabits the vagina is *Lactobacillus acidophilus* which maintains the vagina in a healthy state with its secretions having a pH of 3.8–4.2.

When antibiotics are used for an infection in any part of the body, they often destroy the *Lactobacillus* in the vagina at the same time, resulting in secretions becoming alkaline thus allowing foreign organisms or fungi to grow there. Fungal infections require an anti fungal preparation applied directly into the vagina but bacteria should be treated very differently. The condition of bacterial vaginosis, which causes an offensive, irritating vaginal discharge needs to be treated with an acidifying agent or a vaginal cream of metronidazole (Zidoval) – not with more antibiotics.

After the menopause, the layers of cells forming the vaginal wall undergo atrophic changes because the squamous cells lining the vagina become sparse, dried and decayed and the vaginal wall then becomes thin and lacks elasticity. The collagen tissue virtually disappears, the blood vessels and lymph channels gradually close with loss of blood supply and loss of nutrients, producing a pale, fragile, easily damaged vaginal wall. With loss of blood vessels and loss of collagen from the vaginal wall, the vagina shrinks and loses elasticity and it fails to produce the normal secretions containing the nutrients that can return the vagina to the pre-menopausal state of a young woman. Consequently, the normal organisms that depend on these secretions for nutrients fail to survive, the vagina shrinks, and it becomes painful for a woman to have intercourse. The only way to improve the vaginal wall and restore a healthy environment in the vagina is with estrogen that can either be applied directly to the vagina as a cream or pessary or by circulating in the blood stream.

The **clitoris** is the sex organ of pleasure. A small visible part of it is found in the vulva just in front of the urethra and vaginal openings. The main body of the clitoris is hidden.

The external genitalia are composed of the *labia majora* (outer lips) and the *labia minora* (inner lips). The *labia minora* are designed to close the entrance to the vagina in order to protect it and it also extends forward to form the hood of the clitoris. This visible structure of the clitoris, the glans, is the smallest portion of the total clitoris. The main structure of the clitoris extends from the glans back into the pelvis where it divides to run down the sidewalls of the vagina to end near the anterior wall of the vagina near the junction of the bladder and the urethra, just behind the pubic bone.

The clitoris is anatomically similar to the penis of the male, which extends from the prostate gland at the base of the bladder to the glans at the end of the penis. The cells and tissue that form prostate cells, blood vessel erectile tissue, nerve fibres and excitability of a male penis, are also found in an adult female *within her pelvis* though in differing proportions, and the clitoris responds in the same way to erotic stimulation as does the male penis.

Although the clitoris is the main organ with which females achieve an orgasm during sexual activity, some women obtain intense enjoyment when the deeper clitoral structures near the bladder base are stimulated (the 'G' spot). Even though the clitoris is small, it has thousands of nerve endings that are necessary to convey sensual feelings and responses during sexual activity. During enhanced erotic stimulation, the plexus of blood vessels in the clitoris fill with blood, and the clitoris, like a male penis becomes engorged and erect.[22]

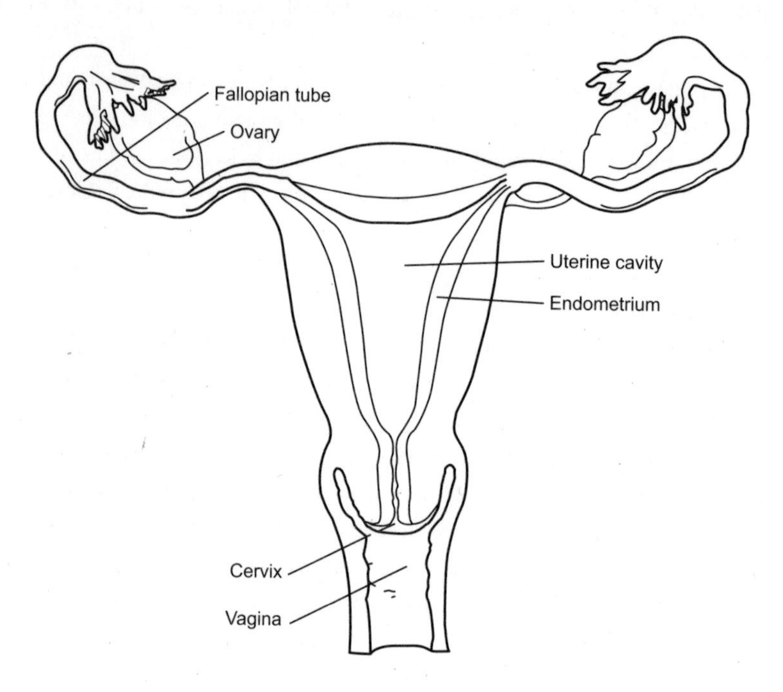

Figure 2. The uterus with the Fallopian tubes.

Ovarian physiology and the sex hormones

Estradiol, progesterone and testosterone are secreted from the ovaries, which lie on either side of the uterus (womb) and these hormones are carried in the blood as it circulates around the body.

When the female fetus reaches seven months of life within the womb, she has two ovaries containing about 7 million eggs. At birth, two months later, the number of eggs has decreased to between 250,000 and 1,000,000 eggs (ova) in each ovary.

By the time a girl reaches puberty at about 12 to 15 years of age, the number of eggs in each ovary has decreased even further to between 50,000 and 250,000. This loss of eggs continues throughout her reproductive years until at about the average age of 50 years, all the viable or usable eggs are depleted.

Sometime between the age of 10 and 16 years the hypothalamus (a complex group of nerve cells in the brain) achieves a level of development that enables it to control and coordinate the hormones of the maturing girl.

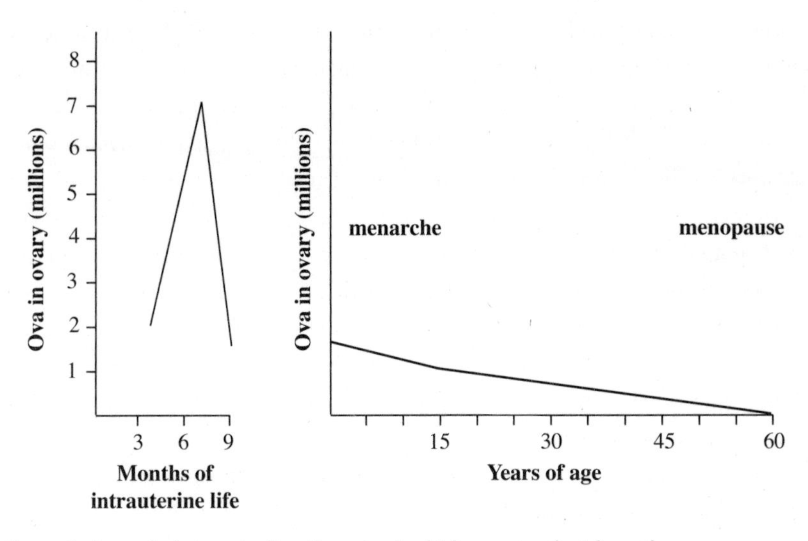

Figure 3. A graph demonstrating the rate at which eggs are lost from the ovary.

The hypothalamus is the automatic pilot of our body. We don't have to think about a number of important body functions that happen involuntarily (such as digesting food, ovulating, sweating, shivering, etc) but these functions are initiated and carried out under the control of the hypothalamus.

The hypothalamus, about the size of a walnut, is composed of bundles of neurons (nerve cells) collected together at the base of the brain, just above the pituitary gland. The neurons have a complex series of connecting nerve fibres, and it is through these nerve connections that they receive necessary information from multiple sites around the body, as well as from within the brain itself. Important autonomous activities are carried out as the hypothalamus responds to impulses or hormone messages. It reacts to a large number of messages such as light, smell (pheromones), sexual stimuli, changes in reproductive organs and the steroids from the adrenal gland, leptin (a hormone produced by fat cells) and angiotensin (a messenger involved in arterial blood pressure), messages from the stomach (amylin and ghrelin) that affect appetite, and to physiological changes to cells within the breast. The hypothalamus also responds to sensations such as heat and cold, body infections, and distribution of fluid within the body. The hypothalamus receives all this information and automatically dictates how the body should respond to these messages. It is responsible for managing and coordinating the cell activity for such important physiological functions as body temperature, water content (thirst), hunger, fatigue, the body response to the circadian rhythm, sleep patterns, sexual desire, ovulation, body maturation and to emotion. When the hypothalamus detects changes in the state of the body it sends messages to subsidiary centres such as the pituitary gland in order to regulate the production of hormones and to maintain homeostasis (harmonious body balance).

As a young girl grows into a woman, her maturing hypothalamus sends messages to the pituitary gland to stimulate that gland to promote activity in the ovaries.

A **gonadotroph** is any hormone capable of stimulating the ovaries or the testicles. The primary gonadotrophic hormone that is released by the pituitary gland is called Follicle Stimulating Hormone (FSH). This hormone is responsible for prompting some of the cells surrounding the eggs in the ovary to produce the sex hormones in order to prepare a young girl for her sexual development, maturation and eventually for a pregnancy.

Under the influence of FSH, cells called **granulosa cells** surrounding specially selected eggs in the ovary, develop the capacity to produce estradiol (an estrogen). When the level of estradiol reaches a certain level in the blood, the hypothalamus recognises this and instructs the pituitary to send a second hormone, Luteinising Hormone (LH), to the ovary in order to induce rupture of the best (largest) follicle in order to release its egg from the ovary.

Following rupture and release of the egg, the follicular cyst collapses like a burst balloon and the remaining granulosa cells form the **corpus luteum** that produces progesterone and also continues to release estradiol. Therefore it is LH that is not only responsible for inducing rupture of the follicle but also to stimulate the cells in the corpus luteum to produce and release progesterone.

To achieve a pregnancy, not only must the ovary produce a viable egg, but if the egg is fertilised, the girl or young woman must have a body and physiological constitution that is mature and capable of sustaining a pregnancy and the eventual delivery of a baby. This is all achieved under the direction of the hypothalamus which, acting through the pituitary, stimulates the production of an ovarian follicle that not only contains an egg but which also produces the necessary ovarian hormones to promote growth and maturation of her body as a girl becomes a young woman.

A young woman produces and releases the very best eggs when she has achieved maturity – usually at about the age of 18 years and her very best years for producing her first child is between 18 and about 25 years. After 25 years of age, the reproductive capacity and quality of the eggs begins to decline until after the age of 35 the *risk* of fetal abnormality due to poor quality eggs increases by about 1 per cent every year.

Estradiol, produced from enlarging follicles in the ovary, induces growth of breast glands and ducts, an increase in size and length of the vagina, thickening and elasticity of vaginal lining (epithelium) and the monthly growth of the lining of the uterus (endometrium).

Progesterone, produced after ovulation in the second half of the menstrual cycle stops endometrial cells from dividing and thus prevents uncontrolled growth. Progesterone also induces a secretory change in the endometrial glands, in preparation for a fertilised egg to implant in the womb and grow into a fetus (unborn baby).

Testosterone, usually thought of as a male hormone, is also secreted by the ovary. Testosterone is responsible for 'igniting' a woman's libido and her drive and her energy – her 'get up and go'.

The combined role of many of the hormones from the ovary, from the pituitary gland and from the hypothalamus is designed to prepare a woman for pregnancy but these same hormones also have many roles other than reproduction. Estradiol is the very potent female hormone which in puberty initiates female characteristics such as breast development, the distribution of female fat (in breasts and thighs), an increase in the size and elasticity of the vagina, an increase in growth of the uterus and pelvic tissue and the maturation of centres in the brain that are responsible for the control and co-ordination of feminine identity and behaviour. Estradiol not only acts on sexual tissue such as breast, vagina and pelvis, but by acting directly on cells, as well as through the hypothalamus, has a very positive influence on bone health and strength, on the heart and arteries, and on the gut and liver, joints, skin, muscles and brain cells.

All these positive actions occur in a young woman as she achieves physical growth, her sexual maturation and her developing potential for reproduction.

During her menstrual life, a woman menstruates about 400 times but usually she has used up all of her thousands of eggs sometime between the ages of 45 and 55 years.

The menopause occurs when a woman runs out of eggs from her ovary. In spite of having hundreds of thousands of eggs available at puberty, the ovary appears to need, and to use, hundreds of immature secondary egg follicles in order to support the one, and sometimes two or three, dominant egg(s) to reach full maturity each time that a woman ovulates.

The end of female production of estradiol and progesterone

During the peri-menopause the ovary gradually runs out of eggs and the amount of hormones secreted by the ovary decreases substantially. However, this loss of ovarian function is not a sudden event (unless the ovaries are removed during surgery or damaged by chemotherapy) but may fluctuate considerably over several years before the menopause. During this transitional phase in a woman's life the level of estrogen may drop by as much as 90 per cent and there may be variable symptoms and bleeding patterns. Because of the irregular and intermittent secretion of estrogen and progesterone by the failing ovary, measuring hormone levels is of little value, but reliance on the woman's medical history and physical examination is of cardinal importance in making a diagnosis of impending menopause. Because the ovary still contains some viable eggs, it is possible for a woman to become pregnant during her time of menopause transition.

Physiological changes during peri-menopause

Estrogen and Anti-Mullerian Hormone (AMH)

Each month many hundreds of eggs in the ovary of a young woman are stimulated to begin the process leading to release of one of the eggs. The recruitment and development of ripening follicles is achieved by FSH from the pituitary gland. As a number of follicles develop they secrete increasing levels of estrogen from the granulosa cells that surround each follicle. These granulosa cells not only secrete estradial but also secrete a second hormone, Anti-Mullerian hormone (AMH). The blood level of AMH reflects the number of eggs in the ovary. When AMH levels fall it suggests that the number of eggs remaining in the ovary is becoming very low. It is now possible to determine whether a woman is in peri-menopause by doing blood tests as she approaches the age when the ovary might fail. When the number of eggs is depleted the granulosa cells are insufficient to maintain normal levels of AMH and the peri-menopause can be said to have begun. The age at which a woman's ovaries are depleted of eggs varies from woman to woman and as a consequence the age at which it is possible to recognise hormonal depletion and its associated symptoms can vary from her late thirties to her mid fifties.

The measurement of AMH levels becomes significant for a woman who has delayed her first pregnancy. Her chances of becoming pregnant are diminished if her blood level of AMH is low, as she may have entered the years of her peri-menopause.

Summary

- Menopause is just one day in a woman's life.
- Menopause is the day that a woman has her last menstrual bleed. It is marked by the end of monthly cycles.
- The menopause usually occurs between the ages of 45 and 55 years and is caused by a woman's ovaries running out of eggs and their consequent failure to produce a woman's sex hormones, particularly estrogen, progesterone and testosterone.
- The menopause is usually associated with the onset of symptoms such as hot flushes, sweats and insomnia.
- The peri-menopause begins when a woman's ovaries begin to fail and the consequent loss of hormones creates many distressing physical, emotional and mental changes.
- The ovaries begin to run out of eggs when a woman is about 35 years of age and this process begins to escalate when she is about 38 to 40 years.
- The peri-menopause is marked by the beginning of irregular bleeding and is complete one year after a woman's last menstrual period.
- The post-menopause begins at the end of the peri-menopause and lasts for the rest of a woman's life. Some symptoms of the peri-menopause, such as hot flushes can continue for the rest of a woman's life.
- Premature menopause is one that happens in the years before a woman has reached the age of 40 years and is believed to occur in 1 per cent of women.
- The human endocrine system maintains the body cells in a stable and functional state of homeostasis or physiological balance.
- The main hormones produced by the ovaries are progesterone, testosterone and estrogen – the most potent estrogen being estradiol.
- A woman's body adapts to changing hormone levels throughout her life but when changes are most dramatic such as during the peri-menopause, she may need therapeutic support to maintain her psychological as well as her physiological equilibrium.
- In Australia, over 3 million women in the population are now post-menopausal.

- Every year between 110,000 and 150,000 women pass from their peri-menopause into their post-menopause.
- At birth a baby girl has 250,000 to1,000,000 eggs in each ovary. At the age of about 50 years all the usable eggs in a woman's ovaries are depleted and the ovaries are no longer able to produce her sex hormones: estrogen, progesterone and testosterone.
- Measuring Anti-Mullerian hormone blood levels is a means of determining whether viable eggs still remain in a woman's ovaries and is therefore a measure of her fertility.
- The menopause for some women, is a physiological, psychological, clinical and sexual disaster which requires understanding and treatment, while other women have no symptoms and feel they have escaped the problems associated with estrogen deprivation, only to fracture bones in their back or hips as they age, or to suffer a premature heart attack, or to experience dementia in their older age.
- The post-menopause is a hormone deficiency state and it is a 'silent' one. It needs to be regarded seriously, discussed fully and managed with empathy and understanding.

CHAPTER 3

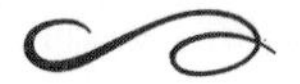

The Women's Health Initiative Study

Early in life, I had noticed that no event is ever correctly reported in a newspaper

—George Orwell

The Study

In 1991, the director of the National Institute of Health in the United States, Dr Bernadine Healy, initiated a large project, The Women's Health Initiative (WHI), with a view to analysing and reporting on the risks and benefits of a variety of strategies that were currently used to influence the health of women after they had passed the menopause. This study is believed to be the largest and most expensive clinical research ever conducted into women's health. (See Appendix 10)

The results from this study have been of immense value in increasing an understanding and appreciation of the events that influence the health and welfare of post-menopausal women, as well as the factors that have a beneficial or an adverse effect on longevity. Part of the WHI Study involved observing the effect of hormone therapy on the health of post-menopausal women and the results obtained from the studies of this group of women are considered in this chapter.

The WHI Study was a Level 1 clinical trial with rigid controls over recruitment of subjects. It was designed to evaluate the risks and benefits of strategies and interventions that could potentially reduce the incidence of heart disease, fractures, breast and colorectal cancer in post-menopausal women. Although it included hormone therapy it was not initially designed to evaluate the benefits and risks of HRT begun as a woman entered her menopause. However, it was anticipated that the results would provide advice and direction to improve the health of post-menopausal women.

Between 1993 and 1998 the WHI Study enrolled 161,809 women. Of these, 16,608 who still had their uterus intact were allocated to receive either Premarin plus Provera or a placebo, while a further 10,739 who had had their uterus removed by hysterectomy, were to receive Premarin only or a placebo.

The women were assessed in 40 clinical centres around the United States where the clinical results were collected by special teams who referred all the data to a group of epidemiologists, statisticians and physicians, at the National Institute of Health for collation, analysis and interpretation. This group, known as the Writing Group, was responsible for analysing and writing all reports on the conclusions reached regarding the results from this large primary prevention study, designed to evaluate the effects of regular hormone replacement therapy in a post-menopausal woman.

To oversee the integrity of the study and to ensure that no adverse effects occurred, an Independent Data and Safety Monitoring Board (IDSMB) reviewed the collected data annually to ensure that the study maintained ethical standards and did not place any woman at increased risk as a result of being involved in the WHI program. At the tenth annual review meeting in 2002, the Independent Data and Safety Monitoring Board was so concerned at the negative aspects reported to them by the Writing Group that they requested the study be stopped. A press conference was called on 10 July 2002 with the express intention of not only halting the Hormone Replacement Therapy (HRT) study, but to advise other women in the United States against continuing their hormone replacement therapy.

On 17 July 2002, the first of many articles written by the WHI Writing Group responsible for collating and reporting on the outcome of the WHI Study investigating the effect of Premarin and Provera on the long-term health of post-menopausal women was published in the *Journal of the American Medical Association* (*JAMA*).[23]

The controversy about estrogen and the use of hormone therapy for post-menopausal women really only began after the press release of the report from the Writing Group who presented data from the WHI Study.

So, what were the results from this huge study, which resulted in estrogen therapy being regarded with such a degree of disfavour? What concerned so many family physicians to consequently develop their insistent and negative opinions about hormone therapy?

Based on instructions from the IDSM Board, the WHI Writing Group reported that hormone therapy increased the risk of breast cancer, stroke, thrombosis and heart attacks and as a result they recommended that women should reconsider any thought of using HRT. During the weeks following the media conference on 10 July 2002, news outlets around the world wrote or broadcast sensational editorials and comments about the adverse outcomes associated with the use of HRT.

The published articles produced a storm of protest from doctors responsible for treating post-menopausal women.

Clinicians (particularly gynaecologists, endocrinologists, neurologists and cardiac physicians) delivered major criticisms of the WHI Study stating that the conclusions drawn from the data were assessed as if all women in the study were of an equivalent state of wellbeing and would respond in the same way no matter what age or length of time since passing their menopause. It appeared that recruitment of women for the study included:

- women who were not seeking hormone therapy;
- women who had already been using hormone therapy for years;
- women who were of inappropriate age to begin therapy;
- women who were considered to be ineligible for hormone therapy because of health reasons; and
- women who did not have menopausal symptoms.

Other criticisms of the study have been levelled at the method of analysis and the unusual presentation of the results. For these reasons it is important to review the structure, the design, the methods and the reason for the curious decision to involve a group of older post-menopausal women in the hormone section of this huge investigation.

Whenever an article is accepted for publication in a medical journal, the authors are usually asked to avoid any particular activity or effort which would suggest that the article contains information or data that makes it more special than other material being published in the same journal. Interested members of the medical profession wait patiently till the journal is published, read the selected article, analyse its contents and then usually make a considered judgment and comment based on close scrutiny of the methods, data, and interpretation of the findings. This time-honoured approach to publication of important results has always allowed specialist scrutiny of medical papers before the media and uninformed health personnel can make hasty and often incorrect interpretation of the results.

However, for a variety of reasons, the presentation of the results of the WHI Study to a select media conference took place one week prior to its publication in the *Journal of the American Medical Association*. This resulted in the media having access to the interpretation of the results and the conclusions drawn up by the Writing Group, *before* any clinicians had seen and analysed them.

For at least one week, headlines in newspapers and other media outlets produced a series of articles and stories presenting grossly distorted opinions about HRT based on the Writing Group's interpretation of the WHI Study results.

In 2006, Dr Karen Swallen of the Centre for Demography and Ecology at the University of Wisconsin-Madison, conducted an academic study in which she reviewed newspaper coverage of the WHI randomised hormone trial.[24] Using the major media newsprint publications in the United States as her source, she found that only 3.0 per cent of newspaper articles provided accurate statistics, most of them failing to include absolute risks, while often including inaccurate relative risks. She found that a number of the articles presented physicians as being ill-informed, out-of-touch or arrogant, and that the pharmaceutical industry was pilloried by the media for encouraging women to use a product that was a major contributor to disease. The pharmaceutical company Wyeth came in for the major criticism in every news outlet.

Dr Swallen commented that most patients rely on their family physician to provide them with advice and information and the family physician depends on medical journals and specialist colleagues to give them guidance. In the case of the WHI Study, neither specialists nor family doctors were given any prior information or access to the WHI Study until after the distorted reports appeared in the media.

It was almost two weeks after publication before medical specialists were able to provide a reasoned and common sense review of the conclusions in the article.

However, the damage had been done.

The suitability of women selected for HRT studies

In spite of pleas to review the conclusions, and the attempts that were made to point out the mistakes and misinterpretations of the methodology of the study (the fact that the women recruited were years too old, they had no menopausal symptoms, many had major medical diseases and many were grossly obese or were smokers), the Writing Group did not retract or change their announcement, and the media proceeded to pursue and highlight the controversy between the concerned clinicians and the Writing Group.

The findings in the published paper and the design of the study, which resulted in clinicians expressing such alarm at the claims that have subsequently been made, were:

1. The trial was specifically designed to determine the risks and benefits of strategies that could potentially reduce the incidence of heart disease, breast and colorectal cancer as well as fractures in post-menopausal women.

(The WHI Study was not initially intended or designed to investigate the influence of hormone therapy on symptomatic post-menopausal women or those who wished to begin HRT. In an attempt to obtain an answer to the question as to whether hormones influenced the health of women, data obtained from older women who had no menopausal symptoms or who did not particularly need or request hormone therapy was included with data obtained from younger post-menopausal women.)

2. Twenty-four per cent of women had been using HRT before they were recruited to the WHI Study.
   (Women who had been taking HRT for up to 25 years would have different outcomes to women who were beginning HRT for the first time.)
3. The women being recruited for the study were required to have no flushes or any other symptoms that are typical of estrogen deficiency. (This was an unusual condition of inclusion in to the study because most post-menopausal women requiring HRT attend their doctor at the time of their menopause because they are experiencing flushes, sweats, insomnia, mood swings, memory disturbance or sexual dysfunction).
   (The study design and subsequent selection of participants for the WHI project would be regarded as completely unacceptable in any institution now seeking to conduct such research.)
4. Some 66 per cent of the participants were over the age of 60 years while 21 per cent were between 70 and 80 years and all were asymptomatic when they were recruited.
   (Most women are between 45 and 55 years of age and usually complain of distressing symptoms when they request to begin hormone therapy.)
5. Beginning HRT ten to 30 years after the menopause is far too late to prevent osteoporosis, cardiovascular atherosclerosis or brain cell damage. This long interval without estrogen for the majority of participants allowed adverse changes to develop in hormone dependent cells before the hormone program was instituted.
   (It is expected that a major difference in clinical outcome will be observed when comparing therapy offered as a preventive measure, prior to the onset of any evidence of a pathological change, compared to the same therapy used to treat a disease which is already producing symptoms – yet the WHI investigators appeared to be unaware of, or to ignore, this as a factor in their analysis of data.)
6. Only 30 per cent of the participants were regarded as being within the healthy weight range while 34 per cent were overweight and 35 per cent were obese. Only 50 per cent had never smoked cigarettes.

(Women attending for treatment as they enter the menopause are generally, younger, fitter, and slimmer and with a better health profile than the older and overweight women who were recruited to the WHI Study.)

7. Some ten days before the first paper appeared in the printed version of the *JAMA* the authors organised a press conference during which the results were released to selected members of the media. At this media 'briefing' the end-points were quoted in relative values rather than absolute numbers (that is, a 26 per cent increase in breast cancer sounded much more impressive than the actual increase of 8 in 10,000, or 1:1250).
   (By presenting their results prematurely to the media in this manner the authors avoided the immediate scrutiny and critical examination normally available to clinicians and other scientists when a scientific paper is published. Apparently designed to attract the maximum attention, this unusual presentation of an article resulted in almost every newspaper and media outlet producing headlines reporting the list of adverse events which, it was claimed, were liable to occur in women who used hormones to treat their menopause symptoms.)

In the week following the extraordinary press conference in which the results were presented to the media, a number of high profile health officials and medical journalists made hasty pronouncements or published some radical opinion pieces in well-known papers.

On 10 July 2002, the health columns in the *Los Angeles Times* and the *New York Times* reported that HRT caused a 26 per cent increase in breast cancer, but the readers were not informed that the actual increase in breast cancer was only 8 in every 10,000.

Women were warned of *an impending explosion in the number of cases of breast cancer among women using HRT*, and the impact on the use of hormone therapy was catastrophic! In Australia, the then CEO of the NSW Cancer Council, issued a statement that all women on HRT should be advised to cease this therapy.

With such high profile organisations and people making such profound statements, it is little wonder that women stopped hormone therapy almost overnight.

Professor Martin Tattersall, oncologist and chairman of the Australian Drug Evaluation Committee that evaluated the significance of the WHI report for the Australian medical community, wrote a reasoned and impartial editorial in the *Medical Journal of Australia* [25] but his report failed to calm the anxiety of women and it did nothing to reduce the alarmist headlines in the media, nor did it affect the attitude of general practitioners who, having read headlines in the media written by health reporters with their interpretation of the WHI Study, followed the advice being expressed by those epidemiologists who were involved in the report.

So misunderstood and aberrant were some interpretations of the WHI results, that some media outlets actually reported that 26 per cent of women who took regular HRT for more than five years would get breast cancer, while others reported that estrogen doubled the risk of Alzheimer's dementia, heart attacks, stroke and embolism.

The use of estrogen therapy to treat symptoms of the menopause was suddenly regarded, not only by women, but also by many in the medical profession, as being inappropriate for management of the menopause. The majority of experts providing such damning commentary on the WHI Study implied, in their comments and advice, that estrogen was the initiator of the increased incidence of breast cancer.

Most of the experts, however, were expert in fields of medicine that are not associated with gynecological endocrinology, and possibly did not have the requisite research background or appropriate clinical experience to interpret the significance of diseases associated with post-menopausal women. Many of them ignored the many glaring problems with the study group. Not only were a large number of the women older (average age 63.5 years) than the usual age group (45–55 years) of menopausal women who consult their doctors about their symptoms, but women with symptoms were excluded, only 30 per cent had a Body Mass Index (BMI) in the desired healthy range (35 per cent were overweight and a further 34 per cent were obese), 36 per cent were being treated for hypertension, 4.4 per cent had diabetes, 12.5 per cent required lipid (cholesterol) lowering therapy and 7.2 per cent had already experienced some cardiovascular accident such as heart attack.

Cardiovascular results from older women (60–80 years of age) using HRT were extrapolated and combined with other results as if they would also be applicable to women 10 to 30 years younger.
(Extrapolating results from a group of older post-menopausal women increases the statistical significance for the total group, but does not make the conclusions clinically valid for younger post-menopausal women.)

A large number of the individual medical outcomes in the WHI study were not significantly different between the placebo and the hormone-treated women, but by using a non-clinical classification called a 'global index' (which clustered all the adverse findings as a single entity) this manoeuvre ensured that negative outcomes were accentuated and in so doing nullified the individual clinical benefits of hormone therapy.

In 2003 the results of a large study called the Million Women Study were published. These results supported the contention that hormone therapy caused breast cancer. The Million Women Study was compiled from a '*cohort study of a quarter of British women aged 50–64 years designed to investigate the relation between various patterns of use of HRT and breast cancer incidence and mortality'.*

In an article in *The Lancet* in August 2003, the senior author of the Million Women Study (MWS) claimed that 20,000 new cases of breast cancer had occurred in Britain as a result of the use of HRT. The National Health Service Breast Screening Program in the United Kingdom invites all women 50–64 years of age to attend for routine mammography. (A questionnaire was mailed to all women who were invited to attend for a mammogram and the self-reported responses from these questionnaires formed the basis of the findings in the published study.)[26]

In 2011 a highly critical review of the series of MWS papers was published. The authors of this critical review wrote:

> *In spite of the massive size of the Million Women Study the findings for the estrogen plus progestogen and for the unopposed estrogen therapy did not satisfy the criteria of time order, information bias, confounding, statistical stability and strength of association, duration-response, internal consistency, external consistency or biological plausibility. If selection bias had altered the identification of breast cancer by as little as 0.3/1000 per year, the apparent risks associated with hormone therapy would have been nullified.*[27]

In the months and years since the initial impact of the WHI Study and the MWS, there has been considerable re-interpretation of the papers and a rational review of both studies is now emerging. Numerous publications criticise the recruitment of an inappropriate group of older women, particularly when data from that cohort is extrapolated as if it was obtained from women entering the first decade of the menopause.[28]

It was as though the epidemiologists responsible for collecting and collating results in the WHI and the MWS Study had trawled through the mass of data looking for associations. When evidence for a relationship was identified the authors appear to have concluded that 'association' meant that a clinical cause and effect existed. In identifying adverse factors in the WHI Study, particular attention has focused on the risk of breast cancer. Following the initial WHI report in 2002[29] involving 16,608 women for 5.2 years it was reported that there was a 26 per cent *increase* in diagnosed breast cancers (from 30:10,000 to 38:10,000 – eight extra cases annually in 10,000 women or 1 in every 1250 women using HRT).

Estrogen was blamed for this increase.

However, a second paper, published in 2004 from the same WHI Writing Group reported on a similar group of 10,700 post-menopausal women who had a hysterectomy and therefore were being treated with estrogen alone (a progestogen is not thought to be necessary if the uterus, with endometrium, has been removed). This time the WHI Writing Group reported that Premarin given by itself for 6.8 years was associated with a 23 per cent *reduction* in the risk of diagnosed breast cancers (a fall from 33 to 26 per 10,000 per year) and blame for breast cancer was then directed towards the progestogen/progestin (medroxyprogesterone acetate – Provera*)* being used.[30]

Neither the expert authorities responsible for the negative cautions associated with the first WHI Study, nor the media, made any significant comment on this second paper reporting a beneficial reduction in the risk of breast cancer associated with the use of estrogen.

In 2011, the WHI Writing Group published a 10.7 years follow-up study on 7645 of the women who had taken Premarin alone.[31] It was found that after almost eleven years the risk of stroke was not increased, the risk of deep venous thrombosis was decreased, the reduction in the risk of heart attacks, bowel cancer and hip fracture was not altered while the risk of a woman developing breast cancer was still reduced by 23 per cent.

Professor Henry Burger, Director of the Prince Henry's Hospital Research Institute, and professor of endocrinology at Monash University, Melbourne, commented on the unusual circumstances in which the initial results were released at a press conference held a week before any health professionals or the general community had an opportunity to examine the data that had led to the dramatic and frightening media headlines. He expressed his opinion 'that the original announcements lacked objectivity and appeared motivated by a strong wish to cast hormone therapy in the worst possible light'.[32]

This point of view was supported in the United States by Professor Bluming, who wrote in *The Cancer Journal:*

> *'... it is difficult to resist the conclusion that the WHI investigators have been doing everything they could to wring the bleakest possible interpretation from their recalcitrant data'. He went on to contend that reports attributing an increased risk of breast cancer, cardiac events and Alzheimer's disease to the administration of HRT required critical review, not blind acceptance.'*[33]

Professor Amos Pines, President of the International Menopause Society summarised the criticism of the WHI Study[34] in the following points:

1. Following publication of the original WHI paper in *JAMA* in 2002, the media and most advisory committees accepted the conclusions as being the definitive report regarding HRT, and it was even suggested by some doctors that all prior clinical trials showing differing results should be downgraded or even ignored.

2. When the WHI Study was being designed, none of the investigators realised or suggested that the age factor was likely to exert a significant influence when determining the consequences of hormone therapy. The cohort recruited was relatively old (average age 63.5 years) with two-thirds being over 60 years of age and only 33.4 per cent being in the age group (50–59 years) considered to be representative of women likely to begin therapy because of menopause symptoms. This important group of young post-menopausal women (only 5522) was too small in number to provide the statistical power to provide the answer to questions regarding the effects of HRT begun at the time of the menopause. Data from the women 60 to 79 years of age was included with data from the younger cohort. No attempt was made to account for the fact that over the 10 to 30 years following the menopause a number of deleterious changes may have already occurred to the cardiovascular system, bone, brain and breast tissue of the older recruited women prior to embarking on the WHI therapy regimen.
3. The data in the estrogen-alone (Premarin 0.625mg) group that reported the benefits of estrogen (such as a reduction in fractures and also of breast cancer) did not receive appropriate recognition or exposure or discussion in medical groups, or in the lay media. This suggests that, as a whole, there has been a deliberate attempt to minimise the benefits of hormone therapy while at the same time, exaggerating the risks.
4. Women should be advised, following a review of all clinical, biological and epidemiological studies over the past 30 years, that they might safely take hormone therapy for symptoms of the menopause. The actual risks are very small while the benefits may be much greater than have been reported by those using selected results in the WHI publications.
5. The selective use of data, and the reporting of statistical analyses in the WHI papers, appears to have been deliberately planned to lead to fallacious and irrational conclusions.
6. Based on the re-analysis of the WHI data, not only by the original authors, but by multiple critics of the findings, the consensus is that the WHI Study requires a completely new evaluation by a team of unbiased experts before any further conclusions can be drawn.[35]

Unfortunate consequences of the WHI Study

When the WHI was published in 2002 and estrogen therapy received such adverse publicity, a very large number of women immediately stopped using HRT in the belief that by avoiding estrogen therapy, they would avoid developing breast cancer.

Ten years later, research confirmed what was feared may occur when a woman stopped her HRT. The Kaiser Permanente Health Organization in Southern California carried out a longitudinal study of 80,955 post-menopausal women. During a mean of 6.5 years of follow up after the release of the WHI findings it was found that hip fractures increased by 55 per cent among those who ceased HRT compared to those who continued on their estrogen therapy.[36]

As estrogen therapy is now known to reduce the risk of atherosclerosis and dementia, an increase in these diseases is expected among the women who stopped their estrogen therapy when the WHI report was released in 2002.

Medical research reports, studies and their interpretations

A Cochrane review is a systematic review of evidence-based medicine with an up-to-date summary of healthcare benefits and risks of a particular procedure or intervention. It is derived from the database maintained by the Cochrane Collaboration *(Archie Cochrane was a Scottish physician who pioneered the idea of Evidence-based Medicine. This concept defines a need for scientific evidence before any new therapy or intervention is instigated).* The Cochrane library online is accessible for anyone, whether a health professional or layperson, to obtain any information to help them make decisions about their own or another's health. The information in this book is drawn from valid scientific research and it can be cross-referenced through an online search of the Cochrane library.

Assessing the quality and relevance of medical studies[37]

Not all studies are equal! Results from medical studies can sometimes be conflicting. Three levels of research are frequently cited.

- Level 1 studies are comparative, prospective, double-blind, randomised, placebo-controlled trials.
- Level 2 studies are observational, frequently retrospective comparison of groups and are not randomised or placebo controlled.
- Level 3 studies are simple reports of cases of treated groups of individuals.
  Medical research studies are explained fully in Appendix 10.

The WHI investigators, in presenting results based on the huge study initiated in 1993, have confirmed that *estrogen plus a progestogen, when begun ten or more years after the menopause* may induce adverse effects to, and be detrimental for the health of older, *at-risk* women.

The same investigators have provided evidence that *unopposed estrogen, begun during the 'window of opportunity' (one to six years after the last menstrual period)* is beneficial, lowering the risk of breast cancer, osteoporosis, bowel cancer and reducing the incidence of calcium deposits in the walls of arteries.

Nearly ten years after the WHI Writing Group released their conclusions following the annual review by the Independent Data and Safety Monitoring Board, a reassessment of the Women's Health Initiative, in presenting multiple papers based on the huge study initiated in 1993, confirms that estrogen therapy, begun during the 'window of opportunity' (the one to six years after the last menstrual period) is beneficial, lowering the risk of breast cancer, osteoporosis, bowel cancer and reducing the incidence of calcium deposits on the walls of arteries, while having no adverse effects on thrombosis, heart attacks or stroke.

The opinion, often expressed by family physicians, that Hormone Replacement Therapy (HRT) is dangerous to a woman's health needs to be reconsidered in the light of recent research and more up-to-date results from the WHI Study, as well as from other significant research.

These more recent large research studies, carried out over a longer period of time suggest that the benefits of HRT far outweigh any adverse events. Even the Women's Health Initiative (WHI) investigators, in a follow-up report in the *Journal of the American Medical Association* in April 2011, (on the estrogen-alone trial of the WHI Study, regarding the health outcome of over 10,700 women followed for over 11 years) confirmed that estrogen reduced the risk of breast cancer by 23 per cent and that the reduction in risk continued for the duration of the study. The same report also confirmed that women who began estrogen therapy as they passed the menopause had a reduction in heart attacks and a 30-40 per cent reduction in bone fractures.[38]

Another major study, which involved 71,237 post-menopausal teachers in California showed evidence of a 50 per cent reduction in the risk of death for women who began hormone therapy as they entered the post-menopause, compared to women who began HRT more than ten years after their menopause. All recent reports on long-term studies, such as the Nurses Health Study, the Kaiser Permanente Study, the California Teachers Study and even including those from the WHI investigators, now confirm that the benefits of estrogen for a young woman, initiated as she enters the menopause, far outweigh any adverse effects which have been identified amongst older women who began HRT more than ten years after their menopause.[39]

Summary

- The Women's Health Initiative Study was a Level 1 clinical trial designed to evaluate the risks and benefits of strategies and interventions that could potentially reduce the incidence of heart disease, fractures, breast cancer and colorectal cancer in post-menopausal women. However, not all studies are equal. Results from medical trials can sometimes be conflicting.
- The WHIM Study, part of the WHI, was conducted to assess the effects of estrogen and progestin on memory in post-menopausal women. The study was flawed because the women chosen for the study were more than ten years older than women who had just passed their menopause and therefore damage to their brain cells had already occurred. (see Chapter 7: Hormones, brain function, memory and dementia)
- The press release of the findings of the WHI Study in 2002 led to controversial opinions being expressed about estrogen and the use of hormone therapy for post-menopausal women.
- A major criticism of the study was the recruitment of women who were unsuitable for the study and therefore the results of the trial were not appropriate when applied to healthy women of menopausal age.
- Other criticisms of the study were levelled at the method of analysis and the unusual presentation of the results.
- Many women stopped HRT and ten years on, research confirmed that what was feared may happen *had* happened – osteoporosis and hip fractures among them had increased by 55 per cent.
- Ten years after release of the misinterpreted results of the findings of the WHI Study, reassessment of the research confirmed that *unopposed estrogen, begun during the window of opportunity (one to six years after the last menstrual period)* was beneficial, lowering the risk of breast cancer, osteoporosis, bowel cancer and reducing the incidence of calcium deposits in the walls of arteries.
- It is essential that the opinion that *HRT may be dangerous for a woman's health* should be reconsidered in the light of a review of research prior to 2002, but also from more recent findings.

SECTION TWO

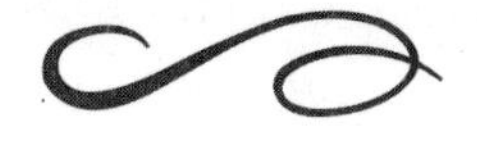

Menopause and Health

CHAPTER 4

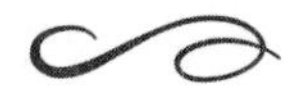

Hormones and genital cancer

Genital cancer is any cancer of the reproductive organs. Genital cancer in a woman includes cancer of the breast, the uterus including the cervix, the ovaries and fallopian tubes, and the genital tract (vagina and vulva).

The cancers that have been associated with the use of hormone therapy (HRT) include uterine, ovarian and breast cancer. (Cervical cancer is caused by a virus – the Human Papilloma Virus (HPV) – or wart virus, and is not affected by the presence or absence of hormones.)

Endometrial (uterine) cancer

In the 1950 to 1960s, when estrogen was first being promoted, it was discovered that the use of unopposed estrogen (that is, estrogen used alone) was associated with an increased number of women complaining of abnormal vaginal bleeding caused by excessive growth (or hyperplasia) of the endometrium (lining of the womb). This excess growth was sometimes associated with an increase in abnormal mutations and genetic changes in the cells in the endometrium, increasing the risk of developing endometrial cancer.[40]

It has been known for over a hundred years that estrogen promotes endometrial cell proliferation in the first half of a normal menstrual cycle and that progesterone stops that proliferation. Unfortunately, when estrogen was first introduced for post-menopausal women, a number of physicians prescribed estrogen alone (commonly Premarin) for these women. This use of unopposed estrogen led not only to hyperplasia (overgrowth) of the endometrium but also to bleeding, and an increase in the incidence of endometrial (uterine) cancer.

In fact, the risk of developing endometrial cancer increased by 1 per cent for every year that estrogen alone was used. This problem was overcome in the 1970s with the simple addition of appropriate progestogen therapy for twelve or more days each month. Progestogen not only stops cells from dividing, but also changes their behaviour from a proliferative pattern to one where the glands and cells stop dividing and instead fill up with secretions (secretory endometrium) in anticipation of receiving a fertilised egg. As cells will only undergo a mutation while a cell is in the process of cell division, the use of progestogens immediately prevented any new uterine cancers from developing.

The use of progestogens in HRT virtually eliminated endometrial hyperplasia, and dramatically reduced the possibility of hormone-induced endometrial cancer[41] to below the rate among women who never used hormone therapy. Today, all hormone treatment programs for post-menopausal women who still have their uterus intact, recommend the use of progestogens for 12 or more days each cycle.

Ovarian cancer

Another major concern about hormone therapy was raised by both the Million Women Study (MWS)[42] in the United Kingdom (which suggested that estrogens increased the risk of ovarian cancer), and the results of the Cancer Prevention Study in the United States that found a two-fold increase in ovarian cancer mortality when estrogen was used for more than ten years.[43]

Publication of these epidemiological reviews once again turned the spotlight on to negative impressions regarding estrogen. However, because ovarian cancer is a relatively rare malignancy (incidence 10.7/100,000 females in the population) and the absolute increase in the number of cancers associated with HRT was very small (1:10,000 per year) the increase was not considered to be so adverse as to significantly alter the positive advice regarding HRT.

The MWS Study suggesting hormones induced ovarian cancer has been criticised because it involved collection of data from women who had multiple variations in their prior history of surgical intervention, variations in the therapy programs being used, differing lengths of exposure time, and lack of consistency in diagnosis, management and outcome.[44]

One of the puzzling aspects regarding the possible relationship of HRT and ovarian cancer concerns the evidence from clinical studies in pre-menopausal women. These studies demonstrate that the use of oral contraceptives composed of the same type of hormones that are used in HRT reduce the risk of ovarian cancer by between 40 per cent and 70 per cent.[45]

Before negative epidemiological studies are accepted as definitive evidence to dictate clinical management, much more research of a biological nature is required to elucidate the action of estradiol on ovarian epithelial cancer cells.

Breast cancer

Breast cancer is recorded as the cause of death of about 4.2 per cent of Australian women. When the Women's Health Initiative (WHI) report was first published in 2002 with epidemiological evidence that women using hormone therapy programs had a 26 per cent increased incidence of diagnosed breast cancer,[46] it was suggested by some clinicians, and publicised widely by the media, that hormones, particularly estrogens, *caused* the genetic mutations in breast cancer.

Risk factors for developing breast cancer

- Family history—two or more close relatives (sisters, mother, aunts, grandparents)—the risk is increased between three to five times
- Age of a woman—the risk doubles every ten years after age 50
- Dense tissue in breasts—risk increased x 2
- Smoking ten or more cigarettes daily—risk increased x 2
- Two or more alcoholic drinks daily – risk increased x 2
- Obesity—risk increased x 1.5
- Sedentary lifestyle—risk increased x 1.5
- Estrogen plus progestogen – HRT—risk increased x 1.26
- Never pregnant—risk increased x 1.2 times
- Prolonged exposure to ovarian hormones—Early onset periods and/or late onset menopause—risk increased x 1.2

No increased risk factors for developing breast cancer

- Only one relative with breast cancer
- History of use of oral contraception

Reduced risk factors for developing breast cancer

- Early age of first full-term pregnancy (18 to 30 years)—30 per cent reduction.
- Breastfeeding for longer than three months—30 per cent reduction

- Estrogen alone as post-menopausal therapy—23 per cent reduction
- SERMs—Raloxifene, Tamoxifen—30–50 per cent reduction
- Tibolone—Livial—60 per cent reduction

Support for the adverse assumption regarding a causal relationship between hormone therapy and breast cancer was followed by a second major epidemiological review regarding the influence of hormones and the risk of developing breast cancer, when the Million Women Study (MWS) was published the following year.[47] The authors of that epidemiological review also intimated that estrogen therapy was responsible for initiating the genetic alterations that caused breast cancer. Hormone therapy had been given bad press and women were concerned that continual use of estrogen would cause breast cancer.

No person or organisation wishes to be accused of endorsing a therapy program which induces breast cancer, myocardial infarction or thrombo-embolism, so, based on the WHI report from 2002, a number of authoritative medical advisory committees were quick to advise women to stop using HRT. A woman who expressed a need or desire to use estrogen therapy was urged to use it at the lowest dosage for the shortest possible period of time.

As a result of the advice from these authorities, and dramatic media headlines, many women (and some doctors) interpreted the WHI Study results as demonstrating that 26 per cent of women using HRT for more than five years would get breast cancer! However, the actual increased risk of breast cancer in the WHI Study was only eight extra cases in 10,000 each year (from 30:10,000 to 38:10,000) or one extra woman in every 1250 women using HRT.

The resultant fear and hysteria associated with misinterpretation of the details and results from the WHI study caused many women to give up their hormone therapy program, while other women deliberately avoided beginning such treatment, even though they were experiencing severe symptoms of the menopause. The fear that HRT caused breast cancer was so overwhelming that it overshadowed the real effects and benefits of using HRT. Women refused to consider its use and family physicians refused to prescribe HRT.

What were the facts and circumstances that led to such panic and to the hasty advice given by various advisers, experts and health agencies?

To answer this question, we need to have a basic understanding of a cancer cell and how it behaves.

Cancer is the Latin word for 'crab'. In early medicine the word cancer was used to describe a malignancy, probably because of the crab-like tenacity that a malignant tumour sometimes seems to show in grasping the tissue that it invades.

Cancer is a disease or malfunction of the genes in a cell. The two main characteristics of cancer are:

1. The uncontrolled growth of cells in the body due to a series of genetic mutations.
2. The ability of these cells to migrate from the original site and spread to distant sites.

The change of a normal breast cell to a cancer cell usually takes many years, during which time the pathological stages of the alterations in the cell can be identified and described.

Atypia is a pathological term applied to a cell that has begun to alter its appearance, and has lost its functional integrity and its relationship to surrounding cells. In the beginning, a few mutations result in *mildly atypical* cells but as more genetic changes occur and accumulate, the pathological change of a cell produces a more *marked atypia.* Following accumulation of more abnormal mutations, the cell develops the typical appearance of a cancer but because it has been unable to break free of its intercellular binding proteins (immunoglobulins) and basement membrane tissue, it remains as *cancer in-situ* (non-invasive).

Cancer in-situ is a form of cancer that is defined by the failure of the cancer cells to penetrate the basement membrane and invade the surrounding tissue. In other words the cancer cells grow in their normal habitat, but do not have the capacity to invade surrounding tissue. They remain in the site at which they originated, hence the name cancer in-situ. It is believed that not more than 15 per cent of cancer in-situ lesions will progress to *micro-invasive cancer* before becoming ***invasive cancer*** with spread to other areas of the body. More evidence is forthcoming that the vast majority of atypias and cancer in-situ lesions do *not* progress to invasive cancer.[48] (For a more detailed review of cancer see Appendix 9.)

The majority of cells with genetic mutations producing various types of atypia remain confined to an in-situ state unless the immunoglobulins and other cell-to-cell adhesion molecules (such as cadherins, integrins), which tether and secure normal cells in their environment, are also altered by mutations. Even though the specific mutations necessary to induce atypia or cancer in-situ may have accumulated in a breast cell, the genetic alterations which allow invasion and metastasis may never be acquired, nor develop, no matter how long a woman lives.

As a result of improved diagnostic techniques such as digitised mammography, ultrasound, magnetic resonance imaging (MRI), fine needle biopsy and/or core biopsy, more micro-invasive cancer as well as cancer in-situ is being found in both pre- and post-menopausal women

With these new diagnostic tools, an earlier diagnosis of breast cancer was expected to result in a reduction in mortality.[49] However, one of the major outcomes of this intense program with a resultant diagnosis of early malignancy (particularly cancer in-situ) has been an increase in surgical procedures – often with removal of one or both breasts and/or treatment with radiotherapy.

In 2011, a 29-year study based on the Swedish Two-County Trial was published. In this trial, 77,080 women were invited to have regular mammograms every two years in order to detect and treat early stage breast cancer. As a control group to determine whether this aggressive seek-and-destroy approach to breast cancer did reduce the mortality associated with breast cancer, the authors demographically matched 55,985 women who were not offered any special investigation or mammographic screening. From results, it was apparent that more cases of cancer were found among women being screened by mammography than in the non-screened population with an improved survival in those having earlier treatment. After 29 years the death rate in women with breast cancer detected by mammography was 24.6 per cent compared to a death rate of 35 per cent among women not being routinely screened for early signs of cancer.[50] This was heralded as proof that intense surveillance investigation was a major advance in the prevention of death from breast cancer.

However, the authors of a Cochrane review have disputed the claim that through early detection, mammograms are beneficial in reducing the number of deaths from breast cancer. This review concluded that the numbers of diagnosed breast cancer in the Swedish Two-County Trial were falsely enlarged by the inclusion of women who had non-lethal, clinically benign, cellular atypias or cancer in-situ in the positive results of the mammography-screening program.[51]

Not only has the Cochrane review cast some doubt on the claim that mammography lowers the risk of death from breast cancer but a recent review from France also suggested that the use of mammograms resulted in a 28 per cent over-diagnosis of breast cancer in-situ.[52] The problem of over-diagnosis by sophisticated techniques, such as digitised mammograms and MRI followed by unnecessary surgery and radiotherapy of breast cancer, is now causing considerable discussion and debate.[53]

Other reviews of breast screening mammography are now being undertaken with a view to attempting to clarify the benefits and risks associated with conducting routine screening procedures. While claims are constantly made that high quality screening mammography has led to a 30–50 per cent reduction in deaths from breast cancer, there have been a number of instances where women have undergone major surgery, radiotherapy and/or chemotherapy following a diagnosis of breast cancer, only to learn later that the radiological diagnosis was not confirmed by a high quality histopathological (biopsy) examination and that the diagnostic procedure resulted in a misdiagnosis. It is claimed that the problem of over-diagnosis of breast cancer has led to inflated reports regarding the benefits of mammography by as much as 30 per cent and that the reported reduction in deaths due to breast screening programs are possibly exaggerated.[54]

Some breast physicians are challenging the aggressive therapy being advocated for managing cancer in-situ and the previously accepted belief that cancer in-situ inevitably progresses to invasive cancer.[55] It is now believed that at least 30–50 per cent, and possibly as much as 90 per cent of breast cell atypias and cancer in-situ, remain in this non-invasive state during the person's entire life[56] – probably because the genes which maintain tissue integrity and cell-to-cell adhesion, have not been altered by a mutation. It is only when immunoglobulins and cell proteins are damaged or altered by mutations that these cell atypias assume the potential for malignant tissue invasion.

It has been claimed that the apparent improved survival rate following mammogram is due to the surgical intervention of breast surgery being performed on women who had severe atypia or cancer in-situ rather than on invasive breast cancer.

In a Cochrane review of breast cancer in 2009 it was estimated that up to 50 per cent of cancer in-situ would never develop clinical invasion and may even spontaneously resolve without intervention.[57]

Genetic mutations in pre-menopausal women

The more one looks the more one finds.

A mutation, in biology, is a sudden random change in a gene or unit of hereditary material. Mutations may be spontaneous or they can be induced by outside or environmental factors such as radiation, viruses or physical or chemical agents. Mutations will only occur during the process of cell division. It is estimated that in adult humans over one million cells divide every second so it is not surprising that every so often the genetic material in a cell splits unevenly with more protein coding material going to one daughter cell and a little less passing to the other. Many mutations are harmless or even improve the cell structure and function, but some mutations have serious consequences. From early in their life a large number of people in the population begin to acquire abnormal genetic mutations. These abnormal mutations are passed on to succeeding generations of cells where further mutations may continue to develop to corrupt a cell, eventually accumulating to cause harm within its host.

For a disease such as invasive cancer to manifest within a person, about 200 mutations must take place and accumulate before a normal cell acquires the necessary changes that will allow it to become an invasive cancer. These mutations do not occur overnight. Some mutations are inherited, some occur as a result of environmental factors and some occur spontaneously during normal cell division. What is clear is that these mutations gradually accumulate within cells as the individual ages over the years.

Several groups of pathologists in the United States, Australia and Denmark have performed autopsies on women who died from a non-malignant cause, and these autopsy results provide detailed and informative data of the sequence of pathological changes as well as data of the ages of women who develop breast cancer.[58]

Results in the table that follows show that when meticulous pathological examination is performed on all the available breast tissue obtained during autopsies that have been carried out on women who died of causes unrelated to breast disease, that pre-invasive malignant changes ranging from moderate atypia to cancer in-situ is found in over one-third of the breasts of pre-menopausal women.[59]

Table 1: RESULTS OF BREAST HISTOPATHOLOGY OBTAINED DURING AUTOPSIES ON WOMEN WHO HAD DIED FROM A NON-MALIGNANT CAUSE

COUNTRY	YEAR	NO. of autopsies	AGE	NO. of breast cancer biopsy sites	PATHOLOGY	
USA	1985	101	40-70	10	DUCTAL CANCER IN-SITU	3.0%
AUSTRALIA	1985	207	16-97	20	MOD-SEVERE HYPERPLASIA	26%
					ATYPICAL HYPERPLASIA	12.6%
					DUCTAL CANCER IN-SITU	3.0%
					INVASIVE CANCER	1.5%
DENMARK	1987	110	20-54	550	ATYPICAL HYPERPLASIA	12.0%
					DUCTAL CANCER IN-SITU	20.0%
					INVASIVE CANCER	2.0%
		33	40-49		DUCTAL CANCER IN-SITU	39.0%
		18	50-54		DUCTAL CANCER IN-SITU	33.0%

In one study involving 110 autopsies performed in Denmark, 275 biopsy sections were retrieved from each breast of young women (20–54 years of age)

who had died from non-malignant causes or unexplained death. In their detailed and exhaustive investigation of the histopathology of breast tissue, 37 per cent of the women aged between 40 and 54 years were found to have cancer in-situ (early non-invasive cancer) cells present in the ducts of breast tissue while only 2 per cent were found to have invasive breast cancer.

The existence of this huge reservoir or collection of abnormal cells (atypias) in at least 10 per cent and probably as much as 30 per cent of the breasts of young, pre-menopausal women explains why over 25 per cent of invasive breast cancers causing death are detected in pre-menopausal women.[60] It may also be the reason why the use of estrogen, by promoting cell division in the breasts of post-menopausal women, results in an apparent increase in detected breast cancer.[61]

These informative studies can no longer be repeated because of bioethical restrictions. These restrictions have been introduced in order to protect the dead from having any further invasion of their body, unless ordered by the coroner.

Women who are post-menopausal, and who have never used hormone therapy, continue to develop cancer as they age with the rate of cancer doubling every ten years, rising to about 15 per cent of women being diagnosed with breast cancer at the age of 80.[62] This is illustrated in the following table.

Table 2: INCIDENCE OF DIAGNOSED BREAST CANCER IN EACH AGE DECADE

AGE OF WOMAN	INCIDENCE OF INVASIVE BREAST CANCER IN WOMEN OF THIS AGE
20-30	1:2212
31-40	1:235
41-50	1:54
51-60	1:23
61-70	1:14
71-80	1:7

Risk factors associated with development of breast cancer

Avrum Bluming, Clinical Professor of Medicine at the University of California, reviewed epidemiological studies in which associations between possible risk factors associated with the development of breast cancer were analysed.[63] Various hypotheses and factors that were thought to be the cause of, or associated with breast cancer, were listed and the relative risks and quantified value were presented in a table. While major concern has been expressed regarding the significance of hormones and breast cancer, it is of interest to observe that women who smoke more than ten cigarettes daily appear to have more than double the risk of developing breast cancer than women who don't smoke, while the drinking of two or more glasses of wine daily also increases the risk by 100 per cent – both associated with a much greater risk of breast cancer than appears to occur with HRT.

The following table,[64] listing epidemiological reports associating various treatments, life events or occupations suggests that the risk of developing breast cancer when estrogen alone is used, results in a reduced risk, while estrogen plus progestogen, although associated with a marginally increased risk, is less dangerous than many social activities in which a majority of women in advanced societies participate.

Table 3: FACTORS THAT HAVE BEEN QUOTED AS BEING ASSOCIATED WITH AN INCREASED RISK OF DEVELOPING BREAST CANCER

RISK FACTOR	RELATIVE RISK
ESTROGEN ALONE	0.77
BIRTH WEIGHT	1.09
FISH INTAKE	1.14
ESTROGEN + PROGESTOGEN (HRT)	1.26
FLIGHT ATTENDANT (Icelandic)	1.87
FAMINE (HOLLAND 1943-45)	2.01
ANTIBIOTIC USE > 4 X PER YEAR	2.07
2 ALCOHOLIC DRINKS DAILY	2.3
SMOKING > 10/DAY	2.4
WAIST / HIP RATIO > 0.8	3.3
ELECTRIC BLANKET USE	4.9

The risk factors often associated with the development of breast cancer are many, but those listed above are sufficient to illustrate the relatively low-risk relationship between the use of HRT and the development of breast cancer.

Marcia Angell, a former editor-in-chief of the *New England Journal of Medicine*, stated 'as a general rule … we are looking for a relative risk (RR) of greater than three or more' (for a finding to be significant).[65] We can assume from such a determination that, of the risk factors associated with the development of breast cancer as listed above, only two relative risk factors – the waist/hip ratio of a woman being more than 0.8 (obese) or the use of an electric blanket are significant, and that the relative risk of the use of estrogen alone or combined HRT is insignificant.

Cluster cancers

Cluster Cancers are cancers that occur in a significant number of people who associate in closely connected communities such as a workplace or geographical area.

While a large number of abnormal mutations may be inherited or occur spontaneously during cell division, there is also considerable evidence that a virus (similar to the already identified Mouse Mammary Tumor Virus – MMTV) may be involved in initiating damage to the balanced genetic working of a breast cell.[66] The presence of a virus (a mammary tumour virus) would explain those instances of cluster cancers that are often recorded in closely associated communities. In 2006, it was reported that thirteen women from a small staff in a television studio in Brisbane were diagnosed with breast cancer during a 12-year period of time. The risk of such a cluster occurring was estimated to be one in a million and while many causes, including irradiation, were suggested to account for such a large number of breast cancers in the one work environment, no cause was identified. Although a virus has not been identified, such a causative factor is considered possible.

Breast cancer is caused by the accumulation of up to 200 abnormal gene mutations, some of which are inherited, some of which occur as a result of chemicals, irradiation or viruses and some of which occur spontaneously as cells are undergoing division.

Estrogen does not cause mutations but may accelerate the growth of a cell that has already accumulated some of the mutations if the cell contains a receptor for estrogen. This is known as an estrogen dependent cancer. At least one-third of all women have acquired a large number of the genetic mutations involved in breast cancer prior to the menopause, while over a quarter of breast cancers are diagnosed in pre-menopausal women.

For a detailed explanation of the influence of hormones on cancer, see Appendix 9.

Summary

- Genital cancer is any cancer of the reproductive organs. In a woman this includes her breasts as well as her pelvic organs – her uterus including the cervix, ovaries and fallopian tubes and the genital tract, which includes the vagina and vulva.
- Cancer of the cervix is caused by a virus.

- Breast cancer is caused by an accumulation of up to 200 abnormal mutations of genes within the cell and the majority of these mutations probably occur prior to the menopause.
- Estrogen does not cause mutations but may accelerate the growth of a cell that has already accumulated some of the mutations if the cell contains a receptor for estrogen.
- Cluster cancers occur in closely connected communities such as a workplace or geographical area suggesting that these cancers may be caused by a virus.
- Other factors such as smoking or the consumption of more than two alcoholic drinks daily have been quoted as being associated with the development of breast cancer.
- A quarter of breast cancer cases are diagnosed in pre-menopausal woman.
- A risk factor for breast cancer is the age of a woman. After the age of 50 the risk of developing breast cancer doubles every ten years regardless of whether the woman has had estrogen therapy or not.
- The findings of the WHI Study released in 2002 that suggested that estrogen causes breast cancer have been seriously questioned, with reassessment of the findings suggesting that estrogen is *not* the cause of breast cancer.

CHAPTER 5

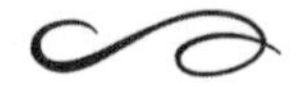

Estrogen and the cardiovascular system

We don't stop playing because we grow old. We grow old because we stop playing.

—George Bernard Shaw

Estrogen is responsible for activating the cells lining the arteries to induce the protective processes that reduce cardiovascular disease. It achieves this by inhibiting the deposition of cholesterol in arteries; by maintaining the integrity of the endothelium that produces the vaso-dilating agent, nitric oxide; and by increasing the production of cholesterol receptors in the liver so that the liver can remove cholesterol from the blood.

As we age, arteries carrying blood from the heart to other organs in our body become stiffer and less expandable and are liable to clog up with blood clots. The stiffness is due to atherosclerosis (cholesterol deposited in the wall of the artery) while the blood clot develops because the endothelium (the cells that line the artery) becomes roughened by the plaques of cholesterol.

Women have a major cardiovascular advantage over men of the same age, both prior to, and during the first decade after the menopause. In Australia and other advanced countries, cardiovascular disease is the cause of death of between 30 per cent and 35 per cent of women. Heart attacks and stroke account for the majority of these.

Fewer women between the ages 40–60 years die from, or suffer from, heart attacks or stroke than do men of the same age.

Death from cardiovascular disease (CVD) in men in Australia is 172 in 100,000 whereas in women, death from CVD is 137 in 100,000. At the age of 50, the incidence of cardiovascular-related death in men is almost twice as high as for women of the same age.

So what is responsible for this protective effect for women?

This difference is due to estrogen, produced in a woman's ovary, acting on the endothelial cells lining the arteries.[67]

The initiating pathological change increasing heart attacks and stroke is usually atherosclerosis or hypertension. Any intervention that has a beneficial effect on these two factors is therefore likely to result in a reduction in premature death.

Following the menopause (but some ten years later than in a man), the risk of death for a woman from cardiovascular disease begins to increase in parallel to the cardiovascular death rate evident in men suggesting that when a woman eventually loses the protection of estrogen, she will experience the same adverse pathological changes as those that develop in a man.

A study of 184,000 Swedish women who had had a hysterectomy revealed that the women who had their ovaries removed with the uterus before the age of 50 years had an almost 40 per cent increased risk of stroke or heart attacks compared to women who had a hysterectomy but whose ovaries were not removed. This suggests that estrogen from the retained ovaries provided considerable protection to the arteries and heart of the women, at least until a few years after they reached the time of their natural menopause. This protection was lost when the ovaries were removed with the uterus. Among the women who were given estrogen immediately following their hysterectomy, the risk of cardiovascular accidents was reduced to normal levels.[68]

To determine whether estrogen does convey a benefit for women, a number of animal studies[69] as well as observational and cohort studies[70] have been conducted which clearly confirm that estrogen, begun at the time of the menopause, is associated with a beneficial effect on the cardiovascular system.

Multiple research papers over the past 60 years have confirmed that estrogen is not only associated with a reduction in the deposition of cholesterol plaques in the endothelial cells (cells lining blood vessels), it also produces an increase in the elasticity and vaso-dilatation of arteries resulting in a lowering of blood pressure in the arteries. This vaso-dilatation depends on the arteries having normal, intact endothelial cells.[71]

The long-term clinical effect of estrogen, whether produced by the woman's ovary or prescribed as estrogen therapy begun during the peri-menopause or at the menopause is to lower blood pressure, reduce peripheral vascular resistance, to improve heart muscle activity and to reduce the risk of myocardial infarction (heart attack) and stroke.[72]

However, if estrogen therapy is delayed for more than five years after passing the menopause, the protective effect may be lost. This is because this delay may allow atherosclerotic changes to take place within the arteries.

If oral estrogen is used, 90 per cent of it passes to the liver and the risk of thrombosis is increased. This is because *oral* estrogen stimulates increased liver cell activity producing an increase in circulating clot factors. If transdermal estrogen is used, only about 10 per cent of it passes through the liver thereby lowering the risk of clot formation.[73]

After the menopause, a delay of ten years or longer before commencing oral hormone therapy allows time for adverse changes such as atherosclerosis to develop in the endothelium of arterial blood vessels. The association of damaged roughened arterial endothelium in an older post-menopausal woman who has been prescribed oral estrogen therapy, thus increasing the production of clotting factor, may result in an increase in thrombosis causing a risk of heart attack or stroke.

In evaluating a woman's suitability for estrogen therapy, her risk factors for possible atherosclerosis need to be determined by assessing her family history, her age, her blood pressure and her cholesterol levels.

The protective effect of estrogen

An important study of the effect of estrogen on macaque monkeys found that if estrogen therapy was delayed for more than two years after castration, the protective effect on the cardiovascular system was lost.[74] Extrapolating these results to humans suggested that estrogen therapy should be initiated within five or six years of the menopause (the 'window of opportunity') to obtain any benefit.

Clinical evidence from studies of humans supports these findings.[75] When estrogen therapy was initiated within five years of the menopause, studies consistently confirm that post-menopausal women experience a 40 per cent to 60 per cent reduction in the risk of myocardial ischaemia (reduced blood flow to the heart), heart attacks and hypertension.[76]

The beneficial effect of estrogen appeared to be so convincing in reducing the risk of death from heart attacks that it was suggested that if estrogen was so efficient in prevention, it might also have benefit in reversing damaging effects in women who had already experienced a heart attack or had a coronary occlusion.

In 1988, the Heart and Estrogen/Progestin Replacement Study (HERS), a secondary prevention trial was initiated. It aimed to demonstrate that estrogen combined with a progestin prevented further cardiovascular disease in women who had previously had heart attacks or coronary by-pass surgery. In this study in which 2763 women took part, the average age of the women was 67 years, they were mostly overweight (with an average BMI of 29) and they had a history of coronary artery damage. The women were randomly allocated to receive either HRT (oral Premarin/Provera) or a placebo. This was a double blind trial, meaning that neither the women nor the investigators knew who had received the placebo or who had received the HRT. In the first twelve months, the risk of death among women receiving the HRT was 50 per cent greater than those receiving the placebo. However, after 18 months there was no difference in the risk of death, and by the second year there was a trend towards a reduction in mortality among the women on HRT.[77]

In 2012, the results of a very significant long term Level 1 study of hormone therapy administered for more than ten years, showed that women who commenced HRT soon after entering their menopause had a significantly reduced risk of heart attacks, heart failure and death, without an increased risk of breast cancer, thrombosis, embolus or stroke, compared to women who had not used hormonal therapy.[78]

A similar rate of adverse cardiovascular events occurred in the WHI Study among older, hypertensive, overweight (BMI 26–30) and obese (BMI 31+) women who had raised cholesterol levels, who smoked or who had other harmful cardiovascular factors at the time of initiating HRT, suggesting that a woman who had developed arterial endothelial damage prior to beginning oral HRT was at increased risk.[79]

The results from both the WHI and the HERS studies suggest that a woman who has damaged endothelium in her blood vessels is at increased risk of thrombosis from oral estrogen whereas a woman with no evidence of damage, who begins therapy within the first five to six years following the menopause, will gain an advantage to her cardiovascular system following use of estrogen by any route of delivery. The earlier a woman begins estrogen, before any damage has occurred to the endothelium of the blood vessels, the less likely it is that a thrombosis will occur.

When estrogen is delivered by a transdermal route (patch, cream or gel), or by an implant, only about 10 per cent of the estrogen passes to the liver with the majority of the estrogen being delivered to other cells before entering the liver. For that reason, the transdermal route of providing hormone therapy results in less clotting factors being produced and therefore less risk of a clot forming. Transdermal estrogen therapy is, therefore, the preferred method of giving hormone treatment to older women, or to those who have some evidence of damage to their cardiovascular system.

Research in France, confirms that a post-menopausal woman using transdermal estrogen (which avoids stimulating the liver), has no greater risk of developing thrombosis than a woman who does not use any hormone therapy.[80]

Thrombosis (clot)

A thrombosis or clot usually occurs as a result of the presence of one or two or all three of the following changes to the blood circulatory system.

1. Damage may occur to the endothelium lining an artery or a vein. Generally the damage will be caused by some trauma such as surgery, an obstetric delivery or an accident, but it may also be due to long-standing damage such as atherosclerotic plaques in arteries or varicosities in veins. The cells at the site of the damaged endothelium release 'sticky' substances to which red blood cells are attracted and become the place where the clot first forms.
2. Stasis or sluggish flow of blood is also a very significant factor in the formation of a clot. Blood that circulates rapidly within a very smooth-walled blood vessel will very seldom become a clot, but when blood flows slowly and comes into contact with a roughened or damaged endothelium, the red cells tend to stick to it. Slowing of the passage of blood frequently occurs in the veins of a woman who is immobilised in bed or a chair following surgery (such as an orthopaedic operation) or who has delivered a baby. Stasis and slowing of the circulation may also occur in any person who leads a sedentary life or who takes a long journey without any physical activity.
3. The third cause for a clot to develop is an increase in the proteins that cause blood to clot. Normally when a person experiences a cut the blood will clot within 3 to 4 minutes and so prevent life-threatening haemorrhage. Most of the blood factors responsible for a clot to form are produced in the bone marrow or in our liver so anything that increases the production of clot factors also increases the risk of a clot. Pregnancy, by increasing estrogen production is nature's way of increasing the circulating clot factors, in order that a woman does not haemorrhage when the placenta separates from the uterus. Oral estrogen, such as is found in oral contraceptives or HRT, which passes from the gut to the liver can also increase the production of these clotting factors. This is why it is important that if a postmenopausal woman on oral HRT or a woman on a contraceptive pill containing estrogen requires surgery she is advised to cease these estrogen-containing therapies for at least one week beforehand, and that she should be active as soon as possible after surgery in order to prevent clot formation.

Unfortunately, a number of physicians, who having read about the increased risk of both heart attacks and thrombo-embolism with oral HRT, frequently advise a woman to avoid using estrogen at all. *They have mistakenly concluded that the risk of thrombosis applies to all estrogens given by any route (transdermal, implant or oral).*

A recent report from the WHI Writing Group confirms that estrogen, administered to a younger woman from the time of her menopause, does not adversely affect her cardiovascular system, but actually reduces her risk of heart attack and stroke. A recent analysis of 1064 women aged 50 to 59 years who participated in the estrogen-only arm of the WHI Study for 7.4 years, confirmed that estrogen resulted in a lower level of calcified plaque in the arterial endothelium than was found in women taking the placebo (Agatston scores 83.1 vs. 123.1) and as a consequence, there was a reduced risk of heart attacks and stroke.[81]

The Agatston score is named after Dr Arthur Agatston who developed a scoring system to measure the amount of calcium deposited in the coronary arteries. When atherosclerotic plaques develop, calcium is often deposited in the plaque. The amount of calcium detected correlates with an increased risk of thrombosis.

Estradiol is known to enhance the ability of undamaged arterial endothelium (inner lining of an artery) to produce a potent vasodilator called Endothelium Derived Relaxing Factor – EDRF (nitric oxide). The ability of estradiol to initiate the release of EDRF leads to a beneficial dilatation of arteries, a reduction in effort exerted by the cardiac muscle to pump blood around the body, and a reduction in the back-pressure in the left ventricle of the heart. Once the endothelium has been damaged by atherosclerosis, the ability to release the vaso-dilating factor is lost.

The conclusion from the studies and research confirms the current view that estrogen given to women within five years of passing into their post-menopause ('the window of opportunity') results in a reduction in heart attacks and a lowering of blood pressure. A delay of ten or more years may increase the risk of hormone therapy causing thrombosis in both arteries and in veins.

Varicose veins

Some doctors have advised post-menopausal women to avoid HRT because they believe that it causes varicose veins, or that women with varicosities should not have estrogen because it causes a clot. However, the relationship of varicose veins, clots and hormones is complex and requires an explanation of the changes in the anatomy of veins and blood flow before a decision is made regarding the use of HRT.

A number of women develop varicose veins during pregnancy and because pregnancy is associated with up to a hundredfold increase in circulating estrogen and progesterone compared to a woman who is not pregnant, it was assumed that hormones caused these varicosities. We now know that this is not so.

Blood circulates in a system that involves it being pumped through arteries, arterioles and capillaries to our organs and limbs. From there the blood is returned to the heart through veins. Blood that passes through the capillaries into veins in our legs will lie stagnant in the soft walled veins unless contraction of our leg muscles compress the veins to push blood back up our body to the heart. For blood to be returned to the upper body, we rely on physical activity such as walking and running to contract muscles and move the blood in our veins. To make it easy for blood from our legs to reach the upper part of our body, the veins have a series of valves which open in one direction only, and which close when blood begins to flow back. This system works very well in young athletic people but sometimes the valves are incapable of maintaining their integrity and they give way under pressure or are weak due to hereditary factors.

Conditions that increase back-pressure on the valves of the veins include pregnancy and specific work situations such as wicket keepers who squat all day with constrictive pads. The development of varicose veins is often associated with stasis (slowing of blood flow), and when this occurs in a person who has damaged vascular endothelium, it frequently results in an increased risk of developing a clot at the site of the varicosity.

Women who suffer from varicose veins are frequently advised to have the varicose veins injected with a sclerosing substance that causes hardening and damage to the wall of the vein. However, this procedure is intended to produce a clot in the vein, further obstructing flow of blood through it. Because of this obstruction, the end result of injected varicose veins is not only oedema or fluid retention of the feet and lower limbs, but also an increased risk of the clot breaking away as an embolus. When a major vein is obstructed, the blood is required to return to the heart through other smaller veins (the collateral circulation) that must eventually increase in size to accommodate the increased blood flow.

Varicose veins are not caused by HRT.

Summary

- The benefits of estrogen on the cardiovascular system of a healthy woman who begins estrogen within the first few years following the menopause far outweigh any potential drawbacks associated with increased coagulation factors and the risk of thrombo-embolism when hormones are begun later in life.

- The beginning of estrogen therapy during the 'window of opportunity' (five to six years following the menopause) is essential.
- Choosing the correct route for giving HRT is also essential in order to achieve this benefit for the cardiovascular system.
- A woman who wishes to commence hormone therapy after the 'window of opportunity' has passed, should have an assessment of her cholesterol levels and her blood pressure to determine whether it is safe for her to do so.
- Estrogen therapy begun at the time a woman is in her peri-menopause or during 'the window of opportunity' results in a reduction in heart attacks and of stroke.
- Varicose veins are not caused by HRT
- A delay of ten years or longer before beginning *oral* hormone therapy, allows time for adverse changes such as atherosclerosis to develop in the endothelium of arterial blood vessels. The association of damaged roughened arterial endothelium in an older post-menopausal woman who has been prescribed *oral* estrogen therapy may result in an increase in the risk of heart attack.

CHAPTER 6

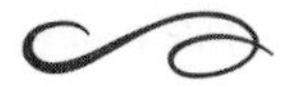

Osteopaenia and osteoporosis

Osteopaenia and osteoporosis are both conditions of degradation of bone due to loss of calcium. As a woman ages she may suffer from bone fractures due to calcium loss and be seriously affected by the disability that results as she is unable to continue her normal lifestyle.

In 2008 *Osteoporosis Australia* issued the following guidelines regarding osteopaenia and osteoporosis:

- ***Osteopaenia*** is the term used to describe a loss of calcium that is so severe that fracture of a bone is possible but has not yet occurred. It is when the amount of calcium in bone is measured to be between minus 1 and minus 2.5 SD below the mean average measurement for a young adult.
- ***Osteoporosis*** is the term used to describe a bone that has loss of calcium minus 2.5 SD or more than the young adult mean.
- ***Severe established osteoporosis*** is the condition that exists when one or more osteoporitic fractures have occurred.

Throughout life, bone is continually being eroded and then rebuilt in a process referred to as modelling/remodelling of bone. The two cells involved in this process are the *osteoclasts,* which eat into and erode bone, and *osteoblasts* that fill in the eroded pits as they restore the strength of the bone. This process is continual and in young people it is responsible for developing the strength and integrity of bone. Bone fragility in older people is the consequence of failed adaptability and defective cell biology, which is the failure of the ageing cell to maintain normal function.

Estrogens are responsible for activating the cells that build and remodel bone. Once bone cells are activated they are enabled to absorb and deposit calcium to produce strong bones. Without estrogen bones may become osteoporotic and may fracture.

Of all reported osteoporotic fractures, 46 per cent are in the vertebra of the spine, 16 per cent are of the hip and 16 per cent are wrist fractures. Approximately two-thirds of all osteoporotic vertebral fractures have no symptoms, but the risk of further fractures is increased *four* times following the first fracture. Women who have had two or more osteoporotic fractures have up to a *nine* times greater risk of a future fracture compared to those who have not had a fracture. This rises to an *eleven* times greater risk if three or more fractures are present. The *fracture cascade* can eventually result in pain, deformity, disability and even early death. Hip fractures are associated with reduced life expectancy. More than 20 per cent of people who suffer a hip fracture (which tend to occur in older populations) die within twelve months, 50 per cent need long-term help with activities of daily living, and 15 to 25 per cent require full-time nursing-home care.

One in three women over the age of 65 will experience osteoporotic fractures.

Calcium is the most abundant mineral in the body. It is needed for many body processes such as blood clotting, release of hormones, and the contraction of muscles. However, if there is not sufficient calcium circulating in the blood, then it is leached from the bones to raise the level in the blood so that the body can function. Healthy bones in both women and men require estrogen. Estrogen, as well as other hormones, activates bone cells to lay down calcium needed for bone strength. If estrogen is not available then the bone cells do not function properly and therefore do not lay down calcium and the bones become osteoporotic.

In 2006, an article describing bone quality involving the material and structural basis of bone strength and fragility was published in the *New England Journal of Medicine.*[82] The authors concluded that the purpose of the continual modelling and remodelling of bone occurring throughout life was to adapt the bone structure to accommodate to the constant changing loads that are placed on the bone as life situations change.

Advancing age results in an accumulation of abnormalities within the extraordinary process that is involved in maintaining the integrity and ever changing pattern of bone strength. For post-menopausal women, factors involved in, and influencing, the intricate bone modelling/remodelling system include hormone deficiency, change to the availability of local growth factors, declining muscle mass and mobility, nutritional deficiency and declining ability to adapt to prevailing loads. The authors of a *New England Journal of Medicine* article concluded that the solution to the problem of osteoporotic fractures involved understanding the cellular processes involved in maintaining integrity of bone in different parts of the body.

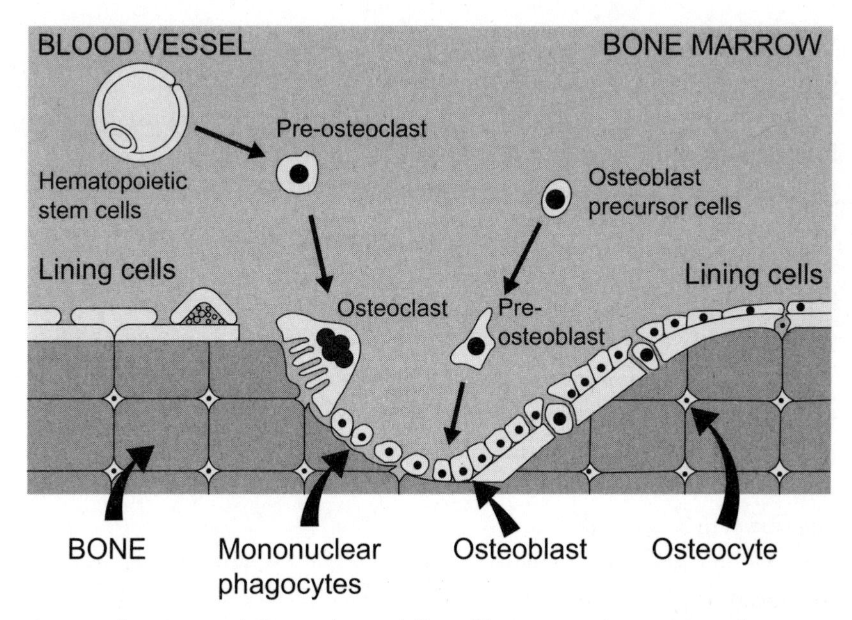

Figure 4. Illustrates modelling and remodelling of bone. Osteoclasts originate from circulating white blood stem cells. They are responsible for eroding 'pits' in the bone. Osteoblasts from bone cells are mobilised to lay down new bone in the eroded areas.

Bone mineral density studies

A bone mineral density study (BMD) is a test used to determine the amount of minerals, mostly calcium, which exists in the bone. It is usual to measure the density of bone in the lumbar spine and in the hip.

It is suggested that a woman who is entering the menopause should have a bone mineral density study (BMD) performed to determine the possibility of osteoporosis developing in the future. If the BMD is within the normal range for a woman of her age, then the next BMD should be performed five to six years later to determine if the loss of estrogen at the menopause has had a deleterious effect on the bone structure and calcium density. If there is evidence of osteopaenia, then active therapy needs to be commenced in order to reduce the risk of fractures in the future.

The BMD is regarded as the 'gold standard' for diagnosing calcium content of bone and risk of osteoporotic fractures. The machines used for this purpose use dual-energy X-ray absorptiometry (DEXA), but different manufacturers supply different machines and as each machine provides slightly different readings, for comparison of the effectiveness of therapy, it is best to have repeated BMD studies performed on the same machine.

Normal bone has a bone mineral density that lies between +1 and -1 standard deviations (SD) of the mean bone mineral density of a young adult.

To reduce the risk of fracture the aim of therapy should be to prevent bone loss before osteoporotic fractures occur or require treatment. With this in mind, it is important to not only maintain the calcium content of bone but also to maintain the bone structure (in much the same way that scaffolding will provide strength and support for workmen while a building is being erected). The use of estrogen, begun at the time that a woman enters the menopause and continued for many years, will prevent the rapid bone loss that can occur in post-menopausal women who have never used or have discontinued hormone therapy. Another significant fact, of which most women are unaware, is that the most rapid bone loss occurs in the first five years after cessation of hormone secretion from the ovary. It is mandatory to begin preventive therapy during the window of opportunity if this bone loss is to be avoided.

The compact outer cortical bone supplies the shape and structure of the bone. Its strength is provided by trabecular bone, which is the scaffolding latticework within the bone. Both the cortical bone and the trabecular bone are responsible for providing the stability and strength of bone. When, as occurs in osteopaenia, the trabecular bone is eroded and the thickness of the outer cortical bone is reduced, fracture is more likely.

While much emphasis in the past has been placed on identifying which site (trabecular or cortical) is most important in causing fracture, it is now thought that both are equally significant. When calcium is lost from either area, the integrity of bone is compromised and fracture may result.

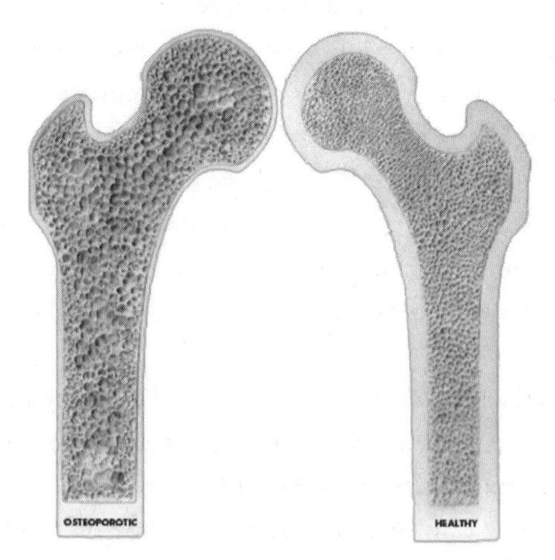

Figure 5. Illustrates healthy bone with dense outer cortical bone and compact inner trabecular bone.

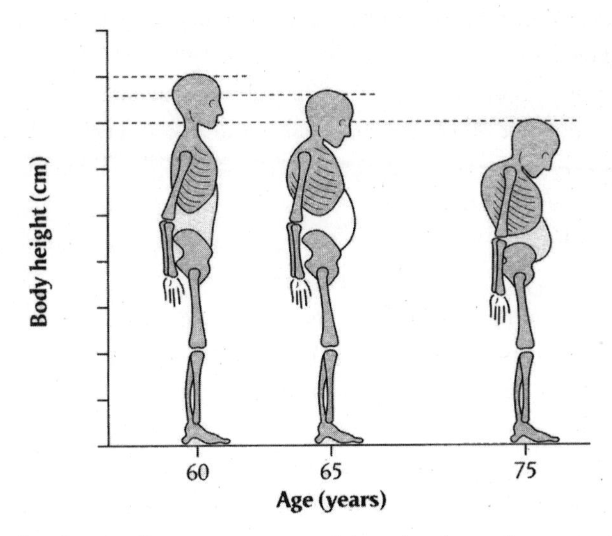

Figure 6. This diagram illustrates curvature of the spine due to the erosion in the spinal column. This particular curvature is known as 'The Dowager's Hump'. As a woman loses calcium from her spinal bones 'crush' fractures of the vertebra can occur, with the most common site being the thoracic region.

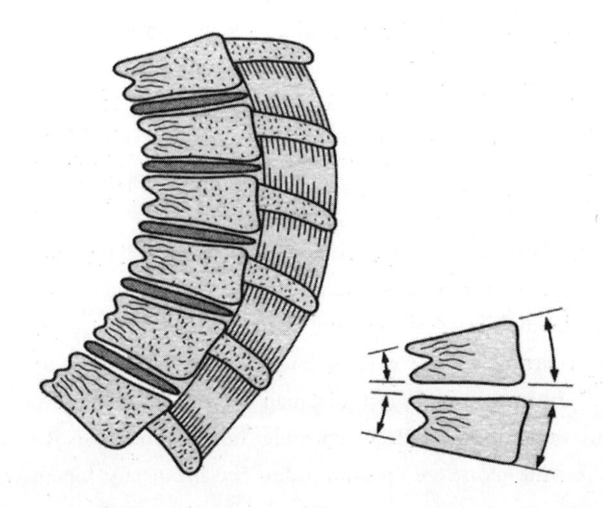

Figure 7. A simple diagram to illustrate that when bone is eroded in the spinal column, it is the trabecular bone in the vertebral body, which is mostly affected.

Bone loss occurs at different rates in different women. At about the age of 35 to 40, some women will begin to lose calcium from bone; it is believed that this calcium loss is related to changes in ovarian hormonal function. The reduction in bone formation probably happens at some time during young adulthood and before menopause.

Following the menopause, some women will lose little more than 1 per cent of bone in a year, while other women are known to lose as much as 10 per cent in that time. The average loss is 2 to 5 per cent for the first three to five years following the menopause but for a woman with a predisposition for rapid bone loss such as heredity factors, her bone loss over a five-year period may be as much as 20 per cent.

Quite often a post-menopausal woman will experience discomfort in her back that persists in spite of rest, physiotherapy, drugs or other treatment. This frequently develops 'out of the blue' with no apparent initiating trauma and is due to a spontaneous crush fracture that occurs when the bone has collapsed in on itself. Crush fractures in the thoracic spinal bones result in the painful and disfiguring change known as the dowager's hump. This begins to be noticeable in women some ten to fifteen years following the menopause and may also be associated with hip fracture following minimal trauma. The simple act of turning over in bed may be sufficient to cause a fracture. It is more important to *prevent* bone loss rather than treating the problem after fractures have occurred.

Various parts of the skeleton lose bone at different rates following the menopause. Some bones, such as the vertebra of the spine, lose a larger percentage of bone than others and this increases the risk of developing crush fractures of the spine before having a fracture of a hip.

By the age of 75 years, almost one-third of women not using HRT will have fractured one or more bones, while over two-thirds will have experienced a fracture by the age of 85 years.

Of the women who are admitted to hospital with an osteoporotic hip fracture, 20 per cent will die within twelve months – mostly due to pneumonia, heart failure and infection due to immobility, bed sores and urinary infection.

Every year in Australia almost 15,000 women fracture their hip and apart from the need for hospital admission and surgery a woman requires rehabilitation, special nursing care and ongoing help after returning home. The costs to the community for hip fracture alone are enormous and the incapacity for an otherwise vital, intelligent and active woman is very distressing.

Osteoporosis Australia has issued a set of guidelines and treatment recommendations for those suffering from osteopaenia in order to reduce the risk of the condition advancing to an osteoporotic fracture. Both men and women should be encouraged to:

- Maintain a good diet.
- Ensure that calcium intake is adequate (800–1200mg daily).

- Ensure Vitamin D levels are adequate (500–1000iu daily).
- Maintain a weight-bearing physical activity (walking for at least 30 minutes every day).
- Ensure that objects likely to cause tripping or falls are removed from the environment.
- Commence appropriate therapy to restore bone strength if bone is fragile to the extent that a fracture is likely to occur, or when fractures have actually occurred.

Therapies for a woman who has osteopaenia/osteoporosis include calcium, Vitamin D, estrogen, bisphosphonates, strontium ranelate, SERMs (such as raloxifene or bazedoxifen) and parathyroid hormone (teriparatide). Because of the cost and the potential for some unwanted adverse symptoms, some of these treatments are not recommended as a prophylactic to prevent calcium loss from normal ageing bone and therefore should be used only for women with severe osteopaenia, bone loss due to cancer, or for a woman who has fractured a bone due to calcium loss.

The role of estrogen in prevention and treatment of osteoporosis

There is a relationship between post-menopausal estrogen deficiency and the development of osteoporosis. Bone cells are 'turned on' by estrogen and even though other pharmaceutical preparations help to reduce the loss of calcium from bone, estrogen is the hormone most effective in maintaining healthy bone cell activity.

Since the 1940s, a huge amount of research has been invested in developing a variety of therapy regimens for treatment of osteoporosis. Estrogen was the first of many regimens proven to be successful in preventing osteoporotic fractures and it is still the premier treatment for reducing the risk of osteoporosis in women. Estrogen inhibits the breakdown of bone and encourages the laying down of calcium, consequently improving the modeling/remodelling process.

Estrogen is the most efficient and cost-effective means of reducing the risk of osteoporotic fractures

In recent years, following the publication of the WHI Study, estrogen has been ignored as the primary treatment to prevent and treat osteoporosis. As understanding of the role of estrogen in the long-term health of women returns, estrogen is beginning to emerge as the best choice to reduce the risk of osteoporotic fractures in women.

The increased risk of osteoporosis for a woman who stops HRT

In 2002, after the publication of the WHI Study, a large number of women who had been using some form of estrogen therapy stopped using it, and concern was expressed that in doing so, these women might actually be placing their long-term health at increased risk. Particular concern was expressed about the cardiovascular system, osteoporosis and dementia. Some women were advised to use a bisphosphonate, or a SERM to prevent osteoporosis, but the majority were advised to use only calcium and Vitamin D.

Ten years after the WHI report, evidence of the incidence of osteopaenia and osteoporosis is now available regarding the effect of stopping HRT, and it does not present a very good picture. In Southern California, the *Kaiser Permanente Health Organisation* has been responsible for the health care of a very large number of the population, including 80,955 post-menopausal women. When the WHI Study became public, the number of these women who used HRT decreased from 83 per cent to 18 per cent and although almost a quarter of the total number of them commenced alternative therapy such as a bisphosphonate or strontium ranelate, the majority did not use any other bone protective treatment apart from calcium and Vitamin D.

At the end of 2008 (six and a half years after stopping HRT), the women were assessed to determine if any fractures had occurred. It was found that their discontinuation of HRT was associated with a 55 per cent increased risk of fracture of the hip while a fracture involving other bones was even more likely to occur. Not only were fractures increased but the longer the time that they were without HRT, the greater the amount of bone was lost. This was evident even among women using other fracture reducing therapy. This study confirms that estrogen is essential for maintaining normal bone structure.[83]

Osteoporotic fractures are a major cause of concern for post-menopausal women – not only because they cause disabling and disfiguring changes in a woman's mobility and appearance, but also because they are a major factor in causing premature death. Efforts to reduce fractures include maintaining the use of hormone therapy, providing sufficient calcium and Vitamin D, encouraging physical weight bearing exercise and ensuring an accident free place to live. If osteoporosis has developed then the use of specific drugs such as a bisphosphonate or strontium ranelate to inhibit further bone loss is recommended.

Estrogen protects a woman against post-menopausal osteoporosis and fractures. Without estrogen a woman has an increased risk of fracture.

Summary

- Estrogen protects a woman against post-menopausal osteoporosis and fractures. Without estrogen a woman has an increased risk of fracture.
- Estrogen stimulates osteoblasts to lay down calcium in bone in order to maintain bone strength.
- Calcium is needed by the body to facilitate muscle function, blood clotting and release of hormones. If the body is not absorbing sufficient calcium for these functions, then it leaches it from the bones to maintain these essential functions. This process increases the risk of osteoporosis.
- Adequate calcium and vitamin D is essential in the diet or as supplements in order to improve and maintain bone health.
- Load bearing exercise such as walking is also required to maintain bone and muscle strength.
- Post-menopausal women can often experience loss of calcium in vertebral bones in their spine, resulting in not only a loss of height as the spinal bones begin to crush, but also a disfiguring dowagers hump. There is also an increased risk of death following the fracture of a hip or some other important bone.
- Thirty per cent of women over the age of 65 years who do not take HRT will suffer from an osteoporotic fracture.
- Almost 15,000 women in Australia will fracture their hip each year and of these about 20 per cent will die within twelve months.
- Any therapy, particularly HRT, which reduces the risk of osteopaenia will result in a lessening of premature death among post-menopausal women.
- If osteoporosis has developed then the use of specific drugs such as a bisphosphonate or strontium ranelate to inhibit further bone loss is recommended.
- Efforts to reduce fractures include maintaining hormone therapy, providing sufficient calcium and Vitamin D, encouraging physical activity and ensuring an accident-free living area.

CHAPTER 7

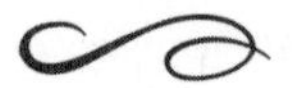

Hormones, brain function, memory and dementia

Dementia is a loss of memory and normal cognitive ability or thought processing in a previously unimpaired person.

In Australia, deaths due to dementia and Alzheimer's disease have more than doubled in the last ten years and account for 7 per cent of all deaths in women and 66 per cent of all deaths due to dementia occur in females.[84]

Dementia in Australia in the year 2010 was ranked as the third commonest cause of death in females, far in excess of genital cancer as cause of death. The following table shows a comparison of causes of death in females:

Table 4

Cause of death	Rank	Total number
Heart attacks	1	10,004
Stroke	2	6,871
Dementia	**3**	**6,083**
Lung Cancer	4	3165
Breast Cancer	6	2840
Diabetes	8	
Bowel Cancer	10	1814
Ovarian cancer		795
Uterine cancer		370

It is known that hormones have a major influence on brain function. Estrogen is responsible for activating brain cells as well as controlling the production of certain neurotransmitters and enzymes that may interfere with, or disturb normal brain function.

Testosterone is also responsible for maintaining and enhancing significant cell activity in the brain, particularly in the limbic system that is concerned with various aspects of emotion and behaviour.

There are several types of dementia with the most common being due to Alzheimer's dementia, to vascular changes, or to toxins.

1. Alzheimer's dementia is probably the most common type of dementia and is diagnosed twice as often in women as in men. It is caused by deposition of a toxic protein called β-amyloid in the neurons of the brain. Over 60 per cent of dementias in women are due to Alzheimer's disease.
2. Vascular causes are most often found in older people and are associated with poor blood supply to the brain due to hypertension, atherosclerosis, small blood clots, etcetera. The result of poor blood supply is lack of oxygen and nutrition to the brain with gradual death of the cells. Between 20 and 30 per cent of dementias are due to vascular disease.
3. Toxic nerve damage such as prolonged use of recreational drugs and alcohol can cause irreversible damage to brain cells.

Impaired memory is a prominent and early symptom of dementia. New skills and knowledge are difficult to learn, while old skills and knowledge are eventually lost. The individual usually has little or no awareness of memory loss or other abnormalities.

Following the Women's Health Initiative Memory Study (WHIM Study), which was designed to determine whether estrogen plus progestin therapy protects global cognitive function in older post-menopausal women, it was reported that post-menopausal women who begin HRT after the age of 65 had a risk of dementia which was twice as great as among women having a placebo.[85] The results of this study of hormonal therapy given to women over 65 years (average age 71) led the WHI Writing Group to conclude that the use of hormone therapy may not be beneficial to women and, in fact, may increase the *risk* of dementia in older women when hormone therapy is commenced *after* the age of 65 years.

There is a difference between *prevention* of a disease and the *treatment* of a disease that already exists.

Using findings from the same group of elderly post-menopausal women (mean age 71 years), the WHI Writing Group published a second article demonstrating that hormone therapy did not improve cognitive function or memory in women aged 65 years or older.[86]

However, as dementia is usually diagnosed in women older than 65 years it is unlikely that prophylactic (protective) treatment begun after the age of 65 years would prevent a chronic disease that has its *origins* in the deposition of β-amyloid in brain cells following the menopause.

In other words, 65 years of age is far too late to begin preventive or prophylactic estrogen therapy.

In the WHIM Study, the hypothesis that HRT given to older women might *reverse* the damage that has already occurred to neurons was being investigated.

As a study in prevention, the WHIM Study was flawed because younger women (50–55 years who had recently entered the post-menopause and who therefore would have gained a benefit from this preventive therapy) were excluded from the study.

Alzheimer's dementia

What are the causes of Alzheimer's dementia and how might estradiol have a positive influence on preventing its development?

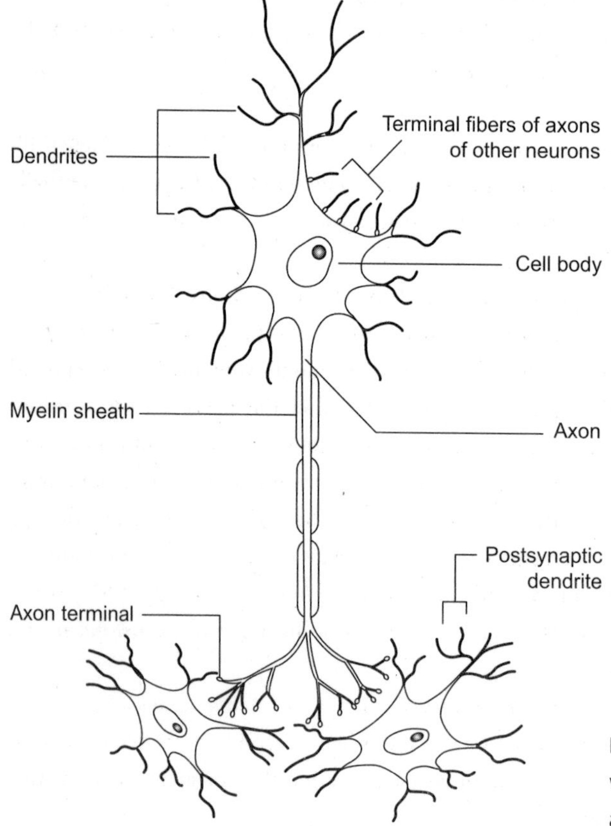

Figure 8. A neuron with dendrites and an axon.

The brain is composed of nerve cells (neurons), which communicate with each other by receiving and transmitting information along thin fibres called nerve processes. Neurons receive information through processes called dendrites and send messages to other cells along processes called axons. A message is transmitted across a gap (synaptic gap) from one cell process to another cell process by chemicals called neurotransmitters. It is thought that on average there are 10 billion neurons in our brain, with each neuron making up to 1000 synaptic connections through the dendrites of each cell.

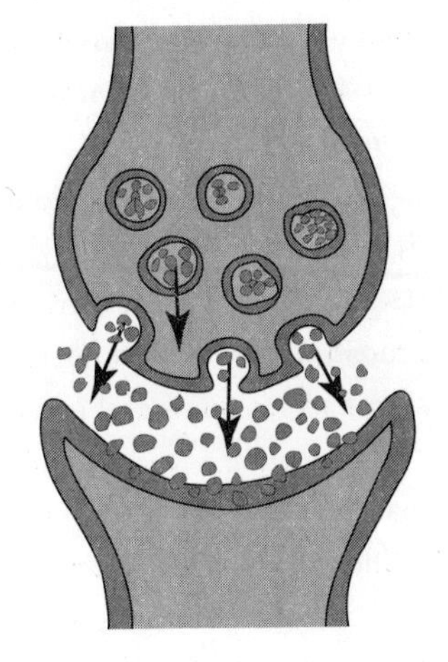

Figure 9. A synaptic junction in the brain demonstrating the release of neurotransmitters.

The **dendrites** are like the tentacles of an octopus that reach out to many other cells in the brain to obtain information, which is then processed within the cell. Each neuron (or brain cell) has only one axon by which messages are sent from the neuron to some other part of the brain or to the body. The message is transmitted to other cells by special neurotransmitter chemicals (such as noradrenaline, adrenaline, serotonin, acetyl choline, glutamate, etcetera) to activate other neurons or cells.

Up until recently, neuroscientists had been unable to determine how each neuron is able to make the right synaptic connection to allow the brain to transmit messages appropriately. Recent research has discovered that neurons produce a specific gene protein at special sites on the surface of the cell that attracts only a dendrite or an axon containing the match for that specific protein. Inability of neurons to produce the specific gene proteins leads to abnormal 'wiring' of the brain circuitry and thus an inability to function normally (autism, dyslexia, etcetera).

Not only do neurons obtain information through dendrites, but hormones and other messengers also play an important role in influencing the function of neurons. All the sex hormones are known to play a role in organising brain cell function and plasticity of neurons but the most significant influence of estrogen and testosterone is found in the different structures and function of the brains of males and females, illustrating how important the sex hormones are in the development and regulation of the central nervous system.

It has long been known that estradiol is one of the hormones that has a major influence on development and operation of the brain, but it is in the possible reduction of dementia that estradiol may play one of its most significant roles for post-menopausal women. It is now known that *Alzheimer's dementia is associated with the deposition of plaques of the toxic protein β-amyloid in the axons of neurons.*

β-amyloid (beta-amyloid) is a toxin that destroys neurons and causes dementia. However, β-amyloid is not normally found in brain cells – it is the result of an enzymatic conversion of a benign precursor called Amyloid Precursor Protein (APP). Within neurons, the APP is concentrated in the synaptic junction site of axons so it is at this site also that β-amyloid accumulates.

Proteolysis is the enzymatic process whereby a complex protein that may be inactive is broken down into simpler substances that often have a high degree of influence and activity on cell function. The proteolysis of the inactive protein APP into the damaging toxin, β-amyloid, is a good example of an adverse cell activity.[87]

Why do women experience Alzheimer's dementia more frequently than do men[88] and why do most cases of dementia in women begin 10–15 years after their menopause?

An enzyme called secretase carries out the proteolysis or conversion of APP to β-amyloid. Estradiol is critical in regulating and suppressing the release of this enzyme. This enzyme, secretase, is responsible for proteolysing (converting) the APP into β-amyloid. Following the menopause, estradiol is not available in sufficient amounts to regulate or suppress the amount of secretase enzyme resulting in an increased amount of β-amyloid being produced. This increase of β-amyloid causes neuronal damage.

Estradiol, by controlling and restraining the release of secretase enzyme regulates and reduces the amount of damaging β-amyloid that can accumulate within neurons.[89]

Also evident in the absence of estradiol, another protein – TAU (which is responsible for stabilising microtubules in neurons) becomes highly degraded (hyper-phosphorylated) by another enzyme (phosphorylase) that is also under the control of estradiol. This process results in clumping of the TAU protein and the development of neuronal 'tangles' with irreversible neuron damage that results in dementia.

Based on this evidence it is probable that estradiol reduces toxic damage to all body cells, but particularly protects brain cells from the effect of β-amyloid and TAU protein, by inhibiting the release of enzymes such as secretase and phosphorylase.

Women who begin estradiol hormone therapy as they pass the menopause (the window of opportunity) have a greatly reduced risk of developing dementia, but if therapy is delayed for several years, the damage caused by β-amyloid and degraded TAU will have already begun and irreversible neurological changes may have already taken place.

In a study published in the *Annals of Neurology in 2010* [90] it was evident that women who began estrogen therapy during the 'window of opportunity' had a 26 per cent reduced risk of developing dementia compared to women who never took estrogens. Women beginning therapy many years after their menopause were reported as having an increased risk of dementia.

Evidence from clinical research studies confirm that approximately 35 per cent of women over the age of 65 will develop evidence of memory loss and dementia[91] – but for women who begin estradiol at the age they pass their menopause, the risk of dementia is reduced to the same incidence as is found among men.

Summary

- Dementia, including Alzheimer's disease, is a loss of memory and normal thought processing in a previously unimpaired person.
- More women than men develop Alzheimer's dementia and most cases of dementia in women begin 10 to 15 years after their menopause.
- In Australia, deaths due to dementia and Alzheimer's disease have more than doubled in the last ten years and account for 7 per cent of all deaths in women.
- Dementia is the third most common cause of death of women in Australia.
- Hormones, including estrogen and testosterone have a major influence on brain function.
- Estrogen is responsible for activating brain cells as well as controlling the production of certain brain neurotransmitters and enzymes that may interfere with or disturb normal brain function.
- Based on evidence to date, it is probable that estradiol reduces toxic damage to all body cells, but in particular it helps protect brain cells from the effect of β-amyloid and degraded TAU protein by inhibiting the release of enzymes such as secretase and phosphorylase.
- Estrogen therapy, if begun in the peri-menopause and during the 'window of opportunity', helps to control the release of both

the secretase and the phosphorylase enzymes that may result in a reduction in Alzheimer's dementia.

- Estrogen therapy started ten or more years after the menopause may actually increase the incidence of dementia by a mechanism as yet little understood.
- The Writing Group for the WHIM study, which was part of the Women's Health Initiative, failed to appreciate the mechanisms involved in brain cell damage, dementia and memory loss, and as a consequence chose an inappropriate group of women to evaluate when considering the possible benefits of estrogen therapy in preventing dementia.

CHAPTER 8

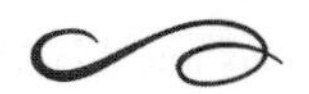

Loss of libido (Hypoactive sexual desire disorder)

The age of a woman doesn't mean a thing. The best tunes are played on an old fiddle.

—Ralph Waldo Emerson

Estrogen, progesterone and testosterone

Low libido (Hypoactive sexual desire disorder – HSDD) is the most common sexual dysfunction experienced by a woman. The problem is not just confined to a group of relatively young women but is a common and distressing symptom for older post-menopausal women and their partners.

The causes of HSDD in older women may include a dry vagina and loss of vaginal secretions; pelvic pain and marked discomfort during intercourse; a decreased ability to achieve an orgasm; loss of sexual desire and even an aversion to sexual intercourse. The presence of such symptoms can cause distressing interpersonal conflict, marriage breakdown, psychological dysfunction, depression and physical harm to the sufferer, with major disruption to family relationships or between friends.

While some women require, and respond well to counselling and other psychological interventions, it is rare for HSDD to be improved by psychiatric treatment alone. Some women may complain of depression as a result of HSDD but most of these women were already feeling unhappy and discontented and they do not improve or respond to anti-depressant therapy.

The main interest from a medical point of view is in the use of hormones and other chemicals to improve and facilitate sexual response and pleasure. There is no doubt that estrogen improves dry, thin, inelastic vaginal epithelium and surrounding pelvic tissue to an extent that pain and discomfort during intercourse is relieved immensely following the start of estrogen therapy.

Estrogen may be administered either by direct application to the vaginal epithelium by using pessaries or creams, or the estrogen circulating in blood which passes through the pelvic organs will have a good effect and influence the cell activity in the vagina, uterus and bladder. The use of adequate estrogen therapy not only improves the sexual tissue in the pelvis and the breast, but also has a beneficial effect on the brain. Some women experience an elevation in mood, lessening of depression and increase in desire following use of estrogen therapy alone, whereas progesterone/progestins in combined therapies may have an adverse effect on mood and libido.

Progesterone seems to depress mood, leading to loss of libido and desire – in fact, high dose progestin therapy has been administered to men to chemically castrate and reduce abnormal sexual urges in those who have committed sexual offences. In a woman it may also reduce sexual desire and cause some psychological symptoms including depression and emotional outbursts in those using various combined hormone preparations containing progestins such as oral contraceptives, HRT, or any therapy that suppresses the ovary.

Testosterone is produced by the ovary and also by the adrenal gland. Androgens produced by the adrenal gland include testosterone and androsterone. After the menopause, testosterone is no longer produced by the ovary but continues to be produced by the adrenal gland. As women age, the adrenal gland also reduces its secretion of testosterone so that the levels gradually decline. Testosterone, amongst other activities, has a direct effect on neurons in the brain and in some women, testosterone has resulted in an increase in motivation, drive, energy and mental clarity as well as a marked improvement in libido.

Female athletes have, for years, used androgenic steroids in order to obtain a physical and psychological advantage over their competitor. It is now also evident that androgens such as testosterone have a major beneficial effect on libido. This is achieved not only directly on brain cells particularly those of the limbic portion of the forebrain, sometimes termed the visceral brain that influences emotional behaviour, but also on the genitals such as the labia and clitoris.

The clitoris is more than the small tip that is situated just in front of the urethra and vagina – it extends back into the pelvis where it surrounds the vagina, and also the urethra near the base of the bladder at what is believed to be the 'G' spot. (Described in Chapter 1). These clitoral cells are similar in function to, and may even be residual remnants of prostatic cells that are so important in arousal and penile erection in males.

Androgens administered for some time are thought to induce these vestigial prostate-like cells to proliferate and thus result in an increase in the sensitivity and ability to respond to stimulation in this area. Adverse side-effects to high doses over prolonged periods of time have occurred, and many female athletes developed acne and unwanted hair growth as well as more muscle bulk. Some of these women also expressed embarrassing sexual urges and it is this effect that has interested the medical profession as a potential therapy for HSDD.

The dilemma when prescribing testosterone for a woman is in determining just how much is needed to achieve a desirable effect without inducing unwanted side effects.

Some studies, using transdermal creams to supply testosterone, have reportedly improved libido, while others using similar amounts of testosterone administered by a different delivery system have found no change. The use of high doses of testosterone delivered by injections for a brief period of time (four to six weeks) will often result in a marked improvement in moods, drive and libido indicating that a woman may respond well to testosterone delivered by a regular cream or implant. If she does report an improvement, then lower amounts of testosterone will often maintain it.

Testosterone cream has also been applied directly to the clitoris and upper labia with the benefit being an increase in the size of the glans clitoris with more intense orgasm.

While other non-hormone therapies and devices to improve libido have been espoused, advertised or sold to women, none of them have been universally effective, and the use of estrogen with testosterone remains the basis of all therapies to enhance sexual responsiveness.

One interesting compound, which is currently being investigated, is an anti-depressant called *Flibanserin* which was originally developed as an anti-depressant drug that acted to block or inhibit the neurotransmitter, serotonin. Women using this compound in a clinical trial to treat depression reported an increase in sexual desire and erotic thoughts. *Flibanserin* is still undergoing trials and is not available in Australia.

While reports such as these suggest that sexual arousal and desire has a neurological basis involving a particular group of neurons which are influenced by serotonin, a remarkable amount of research is required before the particular neurons and region in the brain are identified, and treatment with such drugs becomes available for use as a therapy for HSDD.

Libido (HSDD) is a complex emotion involving interpersonal relationship, desire, pleasure and expectations, combined with physical arousal and the ability to respond. While all these features are part of the complex psychology and the need of individuals, there is no doubt that hormones play a major role in establishing the environmental conditions that ultimately lead to pleasure in sexual activity.

Estradiol is important in enhancing sexual tissue such as breasts, vulva, clitoris and vagina to accommodate sexual activity, while testosterone is responsible for stimulating specific groups of cells in the brain, clitoris and vesico-urethral junction for enhanced responsiveness to sexual stimulation.

Summary

- Loss of libido or Hypoactive Sexual Desire Disorder (HSDD) is the most common sexual dysfunction experienced by a woman.
- Loss of libido (HSDD) is a condition common to women of all ages.
- While some women need and respond well to counselling and other psychological interventions, it is rare for HSDD to be improved by psychiatric treatment alone.
- Loss of libido can be the result of physical conditions that include a dry vagina and loss of vaginal secretions, pelvic pain and marked discomfort during intercourse.
- Estrogen improves and maintains the walls of the vagina and surrounding pelvic tissue thereby relieving pain and discomfort during intercourse.
- Estrogen can be beneficial through circulating in the blood that passes through the pelvic organs or it can be applied to the vagina using pessaries or creams.
- Testosterone can improve libido by acting directly on brain cells in the limbic system that influences emotion and also by acting on genital tissue such as the labia, clitoris and the 'G' spot.
- The use of estrogen with testosterone remains the basis of all therapies to enhance the libido of a woman.

Section Three

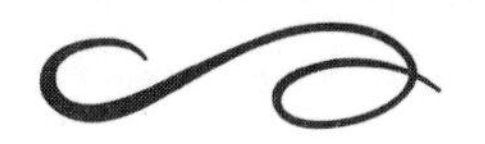

Management of Menopause

CHAPTER 9

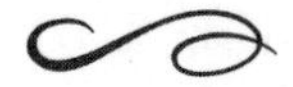

Hormone replacement therapy regimens

Regimen is a medical term that had its origins in the writings of Hippocrates. It refers to a prescribed course of medical treatment, or way of life, or diet for the promotion or restoration of health, or to attain some specific result.

In reviewing the various types of hormone therapies used to treat a woman for post-menopause problems, it is important to consider whether the regimen of therapy being prescribed contains a 'natural' or a 'synthetic' estrogen, whether it should be prescribed in a high or low dose, whether it should be administered by the oral, transdermal, subdermal (implant under the skin) or transbuccal (absorption through the cheek or mouth) route and finally, whether other hormones such as a progestogen, testosterone or dehydroepiandrosterone sulphate (DHEAS) should also be added to the estrogen.

Post-menopause hormone regimens consist of some form of therapy involving an estrogen and/or progesterone/progestin/progestogen or one of the designed chemical agents known as Specific Estrogen Receptor Modulators (SERMs). This chapter reviews regular pharmaceutical hormone compounds as well as commonly used over-the-counter alternative therapy regimens and other products used for managing the menopause.

The development of hormone therapy regimens

In the context of hormone replacement therapy, a regimen is a prescribed program of hormones that is designed to replace the hormones that are no longer supplied by the failing ovaries.

The **oral route** (medication given by mouth) has been the traditional approach when prescribing sex hormones, and it is still the most common method of administering both estrogens and/or progestogens.

In the 1940s, the most frequently used sex hormones available for use by post-menopausal women was either Premarin or synthesised compounds such as ethinyl estradiol and stilboestrol which mimicked the hormones that were released naturally by the ovaries before the menopause.

For the first 30 years, estrogens were administered without the addition of a progestogen, but by the early 1970s it became clear that not only did these unopposed estrogens (estrogen used alone) carry an increased risk of uterine cancer (endometrial cancer increased five- to ten-fold after five to ten years of use)[92] but because oral therapy resulted in about 90 per cent of the estrogen passing directly from the gut to the liver, estrogen was also found to be responsible for an increase in liver cell activity with a resultant elevation of liver proteins such as Sex Hormone Binding Globulin (SHBG) and some of the coagulation factors.

An increased production of liver proteins causes no harm in young, healthy post-menopausal women. Women who are older and who also have hypertension, or high cholesterol levels, or who are obese, or diabetic or are cigarette smokers may acquire damage to the endothelium and the coronary arteries supplying the heart. In these menopausal women who are at risk, the increase in clotting factors caused by *oral* estrogen stimulating the liver raises the chance of heart attacks, stroke or thrombo-embolism.

The Heart and Estrogen/progestin Replacement Study (HERS) study published in 1998[93] confirmed that estrogen, administered by mouth, doubled the risk of a heart attack in a woman who had underlying damage to the arterial endothelium. When the increase in adverse events was identified as being associated with the taking of oral hormone therapy by an at-risk woman, modification to hormone therapies was made to improve both the regimen, and the method of delivery, in order to avoid an increase in cardiovascular problems and thrombosis.

Bio-identical estradiol became the estrogen of choice, while the amount of estrogen that was recommended was reduced to the lowest dose that would control symptoms. Other methods of giving estradiol were developed in an attempt to avoid excessive production of proteins (such as SHBG and clotting proteins) by the liver.

Initially synthetic ethinyl estradiol at 0.5-1.0mg had been used in HRT regimens but this was reduced to levels as low as 0.25mg and finally to 0.1mg before ethinyl estradiol was eventually abandoned in favour of bio-identical estradiol in dosages ranging from 0.5 to 2.0mg. daily. In order to reduce the rate that bio-identical estradiol was metabolised (inactivated by enzymes in the gut and liver), the bio-identical estradiol was conjugated or temporarily fused to another molecule during its manufacture. This process then allowed maximum absorption and circulation of it to cells in the body before it was completely degraded by enzymes.

Transdermal delivery systems were introduced in the 1980s, initially using patches applied to the skin of the lower portion of the body. Estradiol was introduced in an alcohol base in a reservoir patch, which was applied to the lower portion of the abdomen or buttocks for three to four days before being changed. These patches proved to be a great advantage for women who were unable, for various reasons, to take estrogen by mouth.

When reservoir patches proved to be a success, other techniques to enhance the delivery process were explored. **Matrix adhesive** patches were developed containing a variety of doses of both estradiol and a progestogen. These matrix patches were different from the reservoir patch in that the hormone was impregnated in the adhesive, the area in contact with the skin was generally smaller and the adhesive properties were better. It became mandatory to add a progestogen to estrogen in order to reduce the risk of endometrial cancer in a woman who still had her uterus, and a variety of options using progestogens was developed and tested in order to maintain the integrity of the endometrial lining of the womb.

Combined oral estrogen and progestogen regimens came in user-friendly packs and were introduced in order to enable a woman to comply with a correct dose and to ensure that physicians did not unknowingly prescribe irregular or inappropriate doses of hormones. A number of pharmaceutical companies presented their product in these user-friendly packs with a choice of sequential or continuous combined regimens in much the same way that the oral contraceptive pill is packaged.

Although the risk of errors was markedly reduced by these commercial, user-friendly packs, it was also apparent that a major drawback was the lack of flexibility in dose and the inability to vary the estrogen/progestogen ratio. Because of the fixed dosage in these commercial presentations, some women complained of breakthrough bleeding and other problems such as painful breasts and weight gain.

The advantage of continuous combined estrogen and progestogen packs was that after any initial problems, there was a marked reduction in long-term adverse symptoms, a marked reduction in complications such as endometrial cancer and also there was much greater acceptance and compliance of the therapy regimen.

Gels and creams that contain estradiol or testosterone are available for application to the skin and have proven to be very effective and acceptable.

The gel or cream, containing a measured dose of the hormone, is applied to the skin of the lower abdomen or inner aspect of the upper arm (usually at night before going to bed) and the hormone is absorbed during sleeping hours. This transdermal method of application is ideal for women who have developed skin reactions to patches and are therefore unable to use them. Clinical studies confirm this safe and efficient transdermal method of absorbing estrogen or testosterone, but for women with an intact uterus an oral progestogen must also be used.

The search for better, more reliable delivery systems included sub-dermal crystalline estradiol and testosterone implants. While estradiol and testosterone implants are readily inserted and acceptable, it is found that progesterone is almost always expelled within a few weeks.

Sub-dermal implants of pure crystalline estradiol are manufactured in doses of 20, 50 and 100mg for insertion into the fat of the lower abdomen (or the buttock) of a woman who has had her uterus removed. **Estradiol implants** are therefore an ideal hormone regimen following hysterectomy. Implants into the fat of the lower body depend on surrounding blood vessels (capillaries) absorbing a fraction of the crystalline hormone as the blood passes over the surface of the implant. The surface area of the crystalline implant dictates how much hormone is absorbed and the amount delivered daily is similar to that produced by the ovary of young menstruating women.

Progesterone and progestogens (progestins)

Progesterone is required to protect the endometrium of a postmenopausal woman who is having estrogen therapy. Unfortunately, it is one of the most difficult hormones to administer orally in amounts large enough to be capable of providing the protective effect that is achieved by the normal physiological levels of a young menstruating woman. The problem of achieving adequate levels of progesterone is caused by the rapid breakdown of progesterone in the gut and liver.

The failure of progesterone to be absorbed in sufficient amounts through the skin is also a major drawback for the use of bio-identical progesterone in hormone replacement therapy. For this reason synthetic progestogens have been used to adequately protect the endometrium from the proliferative action of the estrogen therapy.

In spite of the difficulty of achieving adequate levels of bio-identical progesterone, it is still regarded as being by far the best hormone to protect the endometrium, without inducing any adverse symptoms. The problem lies in the difficulty of achieving adequate levels.

At present, bio-identical progesterone therapy is not available in an acceptable form and as the amount of bio-identical progesterone that is required to inhibit endometrial proliferation is far greater than can be achieved by the transdermal route, the majority of doctors treating post-menopausal women currently choose to use a synthetic progestogen.

Progestogens/progestins are synthetic products, which have a progesterone-like action on the endometrium. In the United States, these synthesised progestogens are known as progestins but both terms relate to the same synthesised group of hormones. They are usually developed from steroids and they have a configuration similar in structure to either natural progesterone, or to testosterone or to cortisone. As a consequence, the progestogens often have some side effects that may be similar to the effect found in the original compound from which they were derived.

Bio-identical hormones have an identical molecular structure to the hormones produced naturally in the ovary of a young woman of reproductive age. 'Bio-identical' and 'natural' are popular terms used by those who believe that bio-identical estradiol and progesterone is superior to the estrogens and progestogens used in regular commercial HRT. (See Appendix 8)

'Natural' means that the molecule has been derived from a source that has been found in nature. Neither estradiol nor progesterone is found in plants – these hormones need to be synthesised in a laboratory using enzymes to manipulate the molecule from a precursor such as diosgenin that is found in Mexican wild yam or soy. Therefore these so-called 'natural' hormones are actually synthesised bio-identical hormones.

At present, bio-identical progesterone therapy for use in post-menopause regimens is not available in a form which is acceptable to gynaecologists or to the Therapeutic Goods Authority for clinical use, and as the amount of progesterone required to inhibit cell proliferation in the endometrium is far greater than can be achieved by the oral or transdermal route, the majority of doctors treating postmenopausal women currently choose to use a synthetic progestogen.

Most compounding pharmacists dispense bio-identical estradiol, estrone, estriol, testosterone and/or DHEA, either as a transbuccal (mucous membrane of the mouth) troche, or transdermal cream or as a vaginal pessary, all of which are usually compounded in the laboratory attached to the pharmacy.

The hormones being dispensed in compounded prescriptions are promoted as 'natural' and plant-derived and therefore mistakenly assumed to be superior to the hormones used in commercial HRT. What is not mentioned is that the estradiol in regular commercial preparations of HRT is identical to the estradiol in 'natural' bio-identical therapy.

Potent bio-identical estradiol is rapidly broken down within the gut and liver to the weaker estrogens, estrone and estriol.[94] While there is evidence that transbuccal estradiol in a troche will reduce hot flushes and improve the vagina, there is no evidence that estradiol in a troche will prevent osteoporosis, cardiovascular damage or reduce the risk of dementia.

To overcome the known rapid metabolic breakdown of estradiol, pharmaceutical companies have developed a chemical process whereby a stabiliser molecule is attached to the estradiol molecule, thus delaying the enzymatic breakdown process for up to 12 hours, and therefore making it more efficient.

The major criticism of so-called 'natural' estradiol therapy is that the claims of benefits are based, not on research studies involving a 'natural hormone', but on the well-researched results of regular commercial estradiol therapy. *There is no scientific evidence that bio-identical estradiol, in compounded therapy regimens, and prescribed and sold as being 'natural' and therefore different or superior to estradiol in regular HRT, will reduce the risk of osteoporosis, cardiovascular disease, dementia or bowel cancer.*

Another criticism of compounded therapy regimens is that there is no quality control by an independent authority such as the Therapeutic Goods Administration ensuring the safety and integrity of the compounding process (See Appendix 1).

As a consequence of lack of scientific evidence of a benefit, pharmacists and promoters of 'natural therapy' are not legally able to claim that the therapy has any advantage, nor can they include the usual prescriber information inserts about any benefit, or any adverse event resulting from their use. It is the doctor who writes the prescription who is responsible for any claims or adverse events associated with the use of a 'natural' hormone. Therefore, the lack of evidence for a benefit of bio-identical hormones places *legal* responsibility for any mishap regarding the use of 'natural' hormone therapy on the doctor who writes the prescription.

Bio-identical progesterone is thought to be the best therapy to protect the endometrium without producing any of the adverse reactions that have been associated with the progestins in regular HRT. The problem arises with enabling sufficient progesterone to enter the circulation of a woman who still has her uterus in order to inhibit endometrial growth.

Oral progesterone is broken down so rapidly by enzymes in the gut and liver it is difficult to obtain an effective level for clinical use.

Transdermal progesterone has been used, but unfortunately the amount of progesterone being absorbed through the skin is insufficient to have any influence on the endometrium, on a woman's mood or provide any other likely benefit for a post-menopausal woman.

Because of its rapid breakdown by enzymes, bio-identical progesterone was not used for the development of oral contraceptives during the 1950s. Instead, synthesised progestins were used. When post-menopausal HRT was first developed, the synthetic progestins were the obvious choice to protect the endometrium. However, with release of the WHI Study data suggesting that some of the commonly used progestins may be implicated in breast cancer, cardiovascular disease and mood changes, the use of bio-identical progesterone is now being considered.

Various methods of preparation of progesterone have been attempted in order to allow adequate absorption of it without it being rapidly metabolised. The most popular technique currently being used is to crystallise the progesterone molecule and then break the crystals into minute particles so they can be easily absorbed. This micronisation of crystalline progesterone has proven to be effective and an oral preparation (Prometrium) is now available in the USA. Progesterone administered in a troche (lozenge) may result in a reasonable level of it circulating in the blood for up to 4 to 6 hours, but as with all transbuccal therapies, there are no scientific studies to confirm that this method of delivery is effective and safe.

Another method of giving bio-identical progesterone that is being developed is the use of a vaginal pessary or cream containing micronised progesterone. The theory behind this method of giving progesterone is that it is absorbed into the veins surrounding the vagina, and passes alongside the uterus as blood in the veins returns to the heart. Progesterone absorbed from the vagina in this way may be absorbed into the uterus and be sufficient to protect the endometrium before it is diluted and changed during its circulation around the body. More research is required before vaginal progesterone is recommended and becomes available for post-menopausal women.

The use of both bio-identical estradiol and bio-identical progesterone may result in considerable benefit for post-menopausal women if studies confirm that both hormones can be given in appropriate amounts to maintain normal cell activity without causing an adverse effect. The cost for such a research program would be substantial and the time necessary to reach any conclusion would be in excess of several years so it is little wonder that as yet no group, company or government is prepared to fund such an expensive proposal.

Post-menopausal women seeking advice, often scan the internet where there are many articles and advertisements for products and therapies to treat symptoms of the menopause. Some advice comes from respectable medical practitioners, from scientists with a reputation for rigorous scientific research or from medical agencies providing guidelines. Other advice comes from well-meaning friends, hairdressers and pharmacies. Some of the 'advice' offered is developed by some health practitioners who promote their own personal hypothesis or therapy.

It is, therefore, little wonder that many women are confused by these many conflicting ideas and as a consequence often reject all hormone therapy altogether. Some advice available often promotes the use of therapies that not only are of no value but may also cause harm.

Commonly prescribed progestogens that have been scientifically evaluated and confirmed as being of value for use in combination with an estrogen are detailed in Appendix 3.

Testosterone

Testosterone, regarded as *the* male hormone, is a hormone produced in the functioning ovaries of a woman and also in small amounts by her adrenal glands. After the ovaries stop producing testosterone at the menopause, the adrenal glands continue to release it into the blood circulation, but at a diminishing rate. Testosterone improves libido by increasing specific cell activity in the brain as well as increasing the size and sensitivity of the clitoris and the special group of cells surrounding the neck of the bladder known as the 'G'spot'. The 'G'spot is a unique bundle of ducts, glands and spongy cells which, when stimulated in the front wall of the vagina, can enhance the intensity of sexual enjoyment for many women.

Often the level of testosterone circulating in blood will be well within the average range for a woman. However, the measurement of testosterone in the blood alone is not a reliable indication of a woman's need for testosterone. It is also necessary to measure the level of Sex Hormone Binding Globulin (SHBG) which is a protein produced by the liver. If the level of SHBG is higher than it should be, then the testosterone attaches to the SHGB rather than being available for the target cells in the brain, the clitoris and the 'G'spot'.[95] As estrogen increases the cellular activity of the liver, the use of *oral* estrogen increases the amount of SHBG in the blood. As a result, a women taking oral estrogen such as the contraceptive pill or oral HRT often complains of loss of drive, energy and libido associated with her elevated SHBG.

Mainstream pharmaceutical companies have not yet produced testosterone specifically for a woman, so it is prescribed in regimens that are modifications of the male doses and routes of delivery.

Patches and creams may be used to provide testosterone and clinical evidence supports the proposition that these therapy regimens enhance libido. Some pharmaceutical firms have developed creams and compounding pharmacists have dispensed troches to provide testosterone in amounts that increase the very low circulating levels of available testosterone. Injections, implants and oral tablets designed for men are also available and have been prescribed for women wishing to achieve a more positive sexual response to testosterone.

As with any supplement or therapy, it is always a question of balance. If a woman using a testosterone therapy notices or suspects an increase in body hair growth or acne she needs to inform her doctor immediately so that testosterone therapy is stopped until the problem is resolved.

Prescribing advice and HRT

Following the controversy caused by the first WHI Study in 2002, the North American Menopause Society (NAMS) issued a statement in 2010, which encourages caution but advises that:

> *Recent data supports the initiation of hormone therapy at the time of the menopause to treat menopause-related symptoms; to treat or reduce the risk of certain disorders, such as osteoporosis or fractures in select post-menopausal women; or both. The benefit-risk ratio for menopausal HRT is favourable for women who initiate HRT close to menopause but decreases in older women, and with time since menopause, in previously untreated women.*[96]

NAMS also advised that doctors could consider using lower than standard doses of HRT but cautioned that there was insufficient evidence at present to confirm that these lower doses conveyed the same clinical benefit as standard doses of HRT. Some pharmaceutical companies have produced low-dose therapy regimens but data and the conclusions of long-term research into these new doses have not yet established that the low dose is just as effective as 'standard' regimens for all hormone-deficiency problems.

While there may be disadvantages for some women with the use of oral estrogen, there are also some advantages in taking estrogen by mouth, with one positive effect being an increase in cholesterol receptors in the liver. An increase in cholesterol receptors results in an increased uptake of cholesterol by the liver, greater metabolism of blood lipids and consequently a reduction in the damaging low-density lipoprotein cholesterol.

The guidelines issued by NAMS in 2010 are summarised:

1. **Dosage:** Low-dose estrogen and progestogen are capable of maintaining the major benefits of HRT (flushes, sweats, insomnia, dry vagina) while adverse effects are considerably reduced.
2. **Patient advice:** When counselling patients, risks should be conveyed in absolute numbers rather than percentages, to avoid conveying a false impression or inducing unnecessary alarm.

3. **Early menopause:** In women with early menopause, standard dose HRT should be recommended for both quality-of-life issues and for primary prevention of cardiovascular and skeletal bone risks.
4. **Osteoporosis:** HRT may be recommended as a first-line therapy in post-menopausal women below the age of 60 years who are at risk of osteoporosis related fractures.
5. **Coronary heart disease:** Young healthy post-menopausal women can be started on HRT when it is needed without the fear of increased cardiovascular disease risk.
6. **Thrombo-embolism/stroke:** Women who have the potential for, or who have confirmed risk factors for venous thrombo-embolism or stroke, need individualised counselling regarding the risk of oral HRT. It is in these situations, that transdermal therapy (creams and patches) might be preferable to oral preparations.
7. **Testosterone:** Women complaining of distressing low sexual desire and unexplained tiredness or loss of motivation can be counselled about the possibility of testosterone treatment.
8. **SERMs:** There is good evidence that SERMs, which are a specially designed group of medications that act on the estrogen receptors in specific cells of the body, not only reduce the incidence of osteoporotic fractures but also reduce the risk of estrogen-dependent breast cancer. (SERMs are further described in Chapter 12.)
9. **Alternative therapies**: Women who wish to avoid HRT, or for whom HRT is contraindicated, may choose non-hormonal preparations to relieve their symptoms. The degree of symptom relief is much less than is attained with HRT, and there may be unwanted side effects. Long-term safety studies and efficacy trials of most alternative therapies have never been performed and the quality control of them is questionable.

For how long should HRT be used?

Because of the fear that had been created by the WHI report and the MWS results, women were advised to stop using HRT. But some women were so distressed by symptoms that they requested, and often demanded, that their estrogen therapy be continued. Frequently, their doctor would agree to prescribe therapy but only in the lowest possible dosage for the shortest period of time. Such advice was usually based on recommendations from advisory committees who were very conscious of the conclusions that had been published by the authors of both the WHI and the MWS.

The advice usually included statements to the effect that estrogen therapy may be prescribed without causing harm for a period of twelve months, but suggested that it not be used for more than five years.

Why specify these particular periods of time? What would happen if a woman used HRT for six or seven or eight years or even longer?

When considering the reasons to discontinue estrogen therapy the major concern has been that prolonged use would increase the risk of adverse side effects. However, the adverse results for long-term treatment of a young post-menopausal woman beginning therapy at her menopause are few, while the benefits are many. In fact, in long-term studies carried out for periods of time up to 25 years, apart from a marginal increase in the diagnosis of breast cancer, there has been a decrease in adverse effects including a marked reduction in the incidences of heart attacks, bowel cancer and hip fracture. In several of these studies there is evidence that estrogen therapy results in an increase in longevity.

Both the WHI Study and the MWS showed a gradually increasing incidence of diagnosed breast cancers as women continued to use HRT, and this was also evident in both the California Teachers Study[97] that surveyed 56,867 teachers over a period of time longer than 20 years and the Nurses Health Study[98] which had recruited 238,000 nurses beginning in 1974 over a period of about 40 years. The increase in diagnosed breast cancer was highlighted even though the increase was much less than the doubling or tripling effect thought to be of significance, while the reduction in deaths from heart attacks, stroke, fractures, and bowel cancer was ignored.

Salpeter reviewed 19 published articles that discussed the effect of hormone therapy on longevity. She found that the mortality due to heart attacks, colon cancer and hip fracture was reduced to a relative risk of 0.73 in women taking HRT. This compares favourably to the slight increase of death due to pulmonary embolus and breast cancer and the overall health equation for post-menopausal women was in favour of long-term use of hormone therapy.[99]

When considering the reasons to discontinue estrogen therapy the major concern was that prolonged use would increase the risk of adverse side effects. However, the adverse results for long-term treatment of a young post-menopausal woman beginning therapy at her menopause were few while the benefits were many. In fact, in long-term studies carried out for up to 25 years there was no increase in adverse events but there was an increase in longevity with a lower risk of cancer, osteoporosis and heart disease. Both the WHI Study and the MWS showed a gradually increasing incidence of diagnosed breast cancers as women continued to use HRT but there was no increase in mortality in either study. In reviewing the outcome of hormone therapy used as a long-term treatment regimen, instead of a gloomy outlook a quite different picture is seen with fewer deaths and a longer life expectancy.

Most research is conducted by individuals or teams of interested scientists and clinicians who propose a research hypothesis which must be funded, performed, analysed and finally published within a specified time frame. The funding for most research is usually limited to twelve months or five years and the results are usually expressed in these time lines. The WHI Study was designed to last for eight years but was terminated after five years because of the increased incidence of breast cancer.

But was that decision based on reasonable information?

Long-term studies now suggest the advice may have been hasty and actually be counter-productive from a woman's point of view. The famous Leisure World study suggested that women using hormone therapy for more than 15 years did not have an increased incidence of breast cancer while the long-term use of estrogen may have provided women with a considerable advantage over women who did not use estrogen.

The Leisure World retirement village in Southern California has a population of almost 14,000 residents who were all invited to participate in a long-term health review. This review looked at many characteristics of the participants, their treatment options and health outcomes (illness, death, etcetera) and these were recorded annually over the following 25 years. One of the major considerations in this study focused on a review of the benefits and risks of estrogen therapy, Between 1981 and 1985, some 8877 women agreed to enter the Leisure World study into women's health and wellbeing and they became the basis of it.[100] A detailed comprehensive health survey was completed annually for all the women who had agreed to be in the study and the results were published regularly. After 23 years of this ongoing study, mortality results showed that among 4961 women who used estrogen therapy, the risk of death from all causes was reduced by 15 per cent compared to 3840 women who never used hormone therapy. The decreased risk of death was evident for women at all ages.

Hormone therapy used for more than 15 years resulted in a reduction in possible risk of complications of the menopause including osteoporosis, heart attacks, cancer and death and improved the wellbeing of the 4961 women who elected to continue using estrogen therapy. Those who continued to use estrogen over the longest period gained the greatest benefit.

Another long-term study conducted over a period of 17 years also demonstrated that post-menopausal estrogen replacement therapy lowered the mortality rate from all causes of death, but primarily through a reduction in heart disease. The researchers compared 232 women, who began estrogen therapy within a few years of their menopause, with 222 women who never used any hormone therapy. Over 17 years of follow up, the women receiving estrogen therapy experienced a 46 per cent reduction in heart attacks as well as a significant reduction in osteoporotic fractures.[101]

Summary

- Hormone replacement regimens are prescribed courses of treatment to restore and manage the health and wellbeing of women during the peri-menopause and throughout their post-menopause years.
- There are many regimens of HRT available to treat a woman who has passed the menopause and the choice of the route of delivery of these therapies is flexible, depending on the particular circumstances and needs of each woman.
- Considerations for designing a suitable regimen depend on whether the therapy contains a bio-identical or a synthetic hormone, whether is should be administered by the oral (tablet), transdermal (patch), subdermal (implant) or transbuccal (troche) route.
- Post-menopause hormone regimens consist of some form of therapy that uses estrogen, progestogen and testosterone or designed chemical agents such as SERMs.
- Designed to replace the hormones no longer produced by a woman's failing ovaries, the regimen is determined on an individual basis to meet each woman's needs.
- Estrogen may be given to protect the bones and the brain and to improve the vagina, vulva and pelvic tissue.
- Progestogen is given to protect the endometrial lining of the uterus.
- Testosterone is used to improve muscle tone, and enhance the sex organs, the brain and libido.
- SERMs reduce the risk of osteoporotic fractures and also reduce the risk of estrogen-positive breast cancer.
- Evidence suggests that hormone therapy begun at the time of the menopause to treat menopause related symptoms may also reduce the risk of certain diseases such as heart attacks and dementia during a woman's post-menopause years.
- Complementary and alternative therapies (CAMS) are available for women who wish to avoid HRT or for women who are unable to

use HRT, but long-term safety studies and efficacy data on these therapies have never been carried out.

- The use of HRT on a long-term basis is presently being studied. While there is no definitive statement of the benefits of long-term HRT, the Leisure World Study among others is an excellent indicator that estrogen given over a longer period of time may protect a woman's long-term health and wellness and increase longevity.

CHAPTER 10

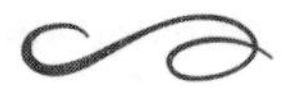

Methods of delivering HRT regimens

There are various means of providing hormone therapies with the most important necessity being to deliver adequate amounts of the hormone to induce a benefit in a specific cell. For example a small amount of estrogen is all that is required to activate the endometrium, but a much larger amount of progesterone is needed in order to protect the endometrium from abnormal change. It is essential when choosing the method of delivery of HRT to not only determine the right blend of hormone therapy but also to understand the way in which each hormone is best absorbed into the body.

Oral hormone therapy regimens

The oral contraceptive pill, composed of a potent progestogen with a synthetic estrogen, was introduced into the Western world in the 1950s. This 'pill' revolutionised contraception and liberated women in terms of their reproductive and sexual life. It had a huge social impact on women – enabling them to gain control over their reproductive capacity and to make choices for their own bodies. It was produced as an easy and convenient oral contraceptive method for all women.

When oral hormone therapy for the menopause was developed it was a natural progression to use the same hormones, though in different dosages, as those used in the oral contraceptive pill. The original method of prescribing HRT was a pill by mouth. The oral method of administration has evolved over the last 50 years and there is now a large range of preparations and packaging using both sequential and continuous therapy regimens. These oral hormone products have been developed following Level 1 studies and are approved for use in Australia by the Therapeutic Goods Administration (See Appendix 1).

Transdermal therapy regimens

The use of the transdermal route as a method to deliver estrogens and progestogens to women was conceived in order to avoid any problems that may occur in association with the oral therapy route of delivery. Because oral estrogens increase liver production of clotting factors that cause thrombosis and raise levels of SHBG, there has been great interest in developing a transdermal delivery system to by-pass the liver.

Bio-identical estradiol and bio-identical progesterone are both absorbed equally through the skin, but because the amount of progesterone required to inhibit the endometrium is 20–50 times the amount of estradiol required to induce growth of the endometrial cells, the use of transdermal bio-identical progesterone has not been accepted as a viable method of treatment. To overcome the problem of obtaining endometrial protection, synthetic progestogens have been used in almost all commercial treatment regimens.

Hormone implants

Estradiol and testosterone hormones have been administered by implants (pellets), which are inserted deep into the fat of the lower abdomen or the buttock. While bio-identical crystalline estradiol and testosterone pellets have been implanted successfully and have proven to be beneficial, progesterone implants are rejected from the body, and are therefore not available for clinical use. If a progestogen is required for a woman who has been given an estradiol implant, then her progestogen must be taken orally.

Estradiol implants: This delivery system utilises bio-identical crystalline estradiol in 20, 50 or 100mg pellets that are ideal for women who have had a hysterectomy and who therefore do not require a progestogen. The crystalline estradiol is slowly absorbed from the implant as blood passes over the surface of the implant. Some implants may continue to release estradiol for up to two to three years following insertion, while the blood level falls slowly as the implant dissolves. The advantage of the implant is that once inserted, a woman does not have to remember to take or apply her hormones on a regular daily or weekly schedule.

The major disadvantages are that insertion of the implant requires a local anaesthetic, and a small incision, while the daily addition of a progestogen by mouth is essential if a woman still has her uterus. If a woman develops estrogen dependent breast cancer after the implant has been inserted, it is difficult to find and remove this source of estrogen.

Implants are usually 'topped-up' every one to two years, but this procedure may be required more frequently if small dosage pellets are used. When menopause symptoms recur, it is an indication that a further implant is needed. However, if the circulating estradiol drops below a level thought to be necessary to sustain adequate cell function for bone and the cardiovascular system (200–400pmol/L) or the level of FSH begins to rise, it is reasonable to insert another estradiol implant without the necessity of waiting for recurrence of symptoms.

[Note: In 2011, the pharmaceutical company producing estradiol implants stopped manufacturing this product. In spite of worldwide protest at the loss of this excellent way to offer bio-identical estradiol, the company has yet to resume production.]

An Australian manufacturing pharmacist has developed a bio-identical crystalline estradiol implant similar to that which was previously available. Crystalline estradiol is compressed in a mould under intense pressure to form a pellet, identical in form and size to the implants previously produced by the original pharmaceutical company (Organon). It contains no excipient, no additives and no binding material. As with the previous implants, it is expected that estradiol will be absorbed from the implant by blood passing over its surface, and this should last a woman for between one and two years before needing another implant. Pharmacokinetic and safety studies are currently being conducted.

Testosterone implants: These are essentially used for men but have been administered to women who experience a loss of drive, energy or libido and who have been found to have a low Free Androgen Index (testosterone/SHBG ratio). There may be a major improvement in wellbeing, drive, energy and libido following the implantation of a testosterone pellet. It is usual to use a testosterone implant of 100mg but, if this dose is considered as too high for a female, it may be broken in half. A 100mg implant will often last for six months before requiring a 'top-up'. The major adverse complication when too much testosterone is administered is hair growth, acne, alopecia and a deep voice but these are uncommon when care is taken when deciding to use testosterone.

Troches

Troches are lozenges, which contain different doses and amounts of bio- identical hormones such as estradiol, oestrone, oestriol, progesterone, testosterone and/or dehydropeiandrosterone (DHEA). Troches are placed in the cheek of the mouth and allowed to dissolve like a lozenge. It takes 20–30 minutes for a troche to dissolve completely. Blood levels of the hormones that are absorbed in the mouth are elevated above physiological levels for a very short space of time, but return to base-line levels within four to eight hours[102] The use of a troche to deliver HRT is controversial because there is no scientific confirmation that it protects bones, the brain or the cardiovascular system. There is no quality control by an independent regulatory authority ensuring the safety and integrity of the methods of preparing troches. The advantage of a troche is that it allows bio-identical estradiol to be delivered at levels that result in control of menopausal symptoms such as flushes and a dry vagina.

Prescriptions for troches are provided by doctors and are often found to contain a mix of hormones. Some prescriptions even include estrone and estriol as well as estradiol (referred to as Tri-est in prescriptions), when it is known that estradiol (the primary, potent estrogen from the ovary) will be converted naturally and rapidly to estrone in the body, and then to the excretory product estriol. Therefore it is not necessary to have estrone and estriol added to a prescription containing estradiol.

Other troche prescriptions may contain Dehydroepiandrosterone (DHEA) or Pregnenolone. DHEA is a precursor metabolite from the adrenal gland and is not a messenger hormone. DHEA can be metabolised by enzymes into hormones such as androstenedione, testosterone and estradiol. Reports of good results from the use of troches containing DHEA is probably due to the effect of this product being metabolised by enzymes to estradiol or testosterone. Pregnenolone is also a precursor derived by enzymatic activity from cholesterol molecules, produced by the liver. Pregnenolone has no action unless other enzymes convert it into active progesterone or androstenedione. Most of these enzymes are found in the active ovary of a young woman, so after the menopause, when the ovary is no longer functioning, conversion of pregnenolone to sex hormones is not possible.

Unfortunately, there has been very little acceptable scientific research conducted by the supporters of troches containing Tri-est or DHEA to substantiate claims for their effectiveness or their safety. Because only small amounts of estradiol are necessary to achieve remission of most menopausal symptoms, and because transbuccal absorption of hormones bypass the gut and liver, the troche is often extolled as being the best delivery system for providing hormone therapy. (See Chapter 13–DHEAS)

While the transbuccal route of delivery may well be advantageous, no research is available which has identified the amount of progesterone that is required in a troche to convert or protect the endometrium from any hypertrophic change induced by estradiol.

The troche may in the future (if properly conducted research confirms the benefits) provide an alternative for administration of hormones for women who prefer to obtain their therapy by a route other than the traditional oral or transdermal approach.

The concerns and disadvantages with this method of medication are:

1. The majority of doctors writing the prescriptions have very little knowledge or understanding of the pharmacokinetics (how the drug is absorbed, distributed, metabolised and eliminated by the body) or the safety profile of the hormones they are prescribing.
2. The prescription for a troche is compounded by an independent pharmacist, and equality of dosage cannot be guaranteed from one troche to the next.
3. There is no quality control that ascertains and guarantees the content and stability of the hormone in each dispensed troche.
4. There is no data to confirm that estradiol delivered in this fashion will reduce the possibility of cardiovascular disease, osteoporosis or dementia.
5. Safety studies have never been performed to ensure that the hormones prescribed in a troche actually achieve what was intended without inducing an abnormal cell response such as abnormal bleeding or cancer of the endometrium.
6. Troches are more expensive than commercially produced hormone regimens.
7. Troches sometimes cause irritation when dissolving in the cheek.

Vaginal therapy

One method that has been utilised for centuries and is still a very acceptable method of administration of a drug, particularly a hormone, is through the vagina. Estradiol is readily absorbed through all body tissue surfaces including the vagina. For a woman who has been treated for breast cancer, and is suffering from vaginal atrophy and marked pain on intercourse, creams and pessaries of estrogens are available.

A pessary (Vagifem) containing 25mcg of estradiol hemihydrate is one form of estrogen that has been developed. Because the dosage is low, the total amount of estradiol absorbed into the blood system is extremely small – for that reason it is often prescribed for women who have a dry vagina but who are unable or unwilling to use regular hormone therapy. Vagifem is normally used twice weekly, but when the vaginal epithelium has recovered moisture and elasticity it may be reduced to once weekly. Vaginal estrogen has no adverse effect on a sexual partner.

Ovestin cream and pessaries: Estriol, the weakest of the estrogens available for post-menopausal women, has a relatively low potency when compared to estradiol and estrone. It may be administered as a cream or as a pessary into the vagina to improve the moisture and elasticity of the epithelium for post-menopausal women who are not able to use regular hormone therapy, or who require pre-operative tissue regeneration prior to vaginal surgery. There is evidence that this method of delivery of estriol is as effective as regular estradiol, given by the oral or transdermal route, in improving the vaginal epithelium.

There are many hormone preparations available to treat symptoms of the menopause and there are also many ways of giving them. Every woman must be given the appropriate information which will allow her to choose the hormone delivery system she could use and what hormones and dose can fulfil her needs.

Summary

- There are different means of providing hormone therapies with the most important necessity being to deliver adequate amounts of the hormones to induce a benefit in a specific cell.
- Oral hormone replacement therapy has evolved as a natural progression from 'the pill', using the same hormones in different dosages. This oral method of having hormone therapy has evolved over the last 50 years and there is now a large range of commercial HRT preparations and user-friendly packs providing both sequential and continuous therapy regimens.
- The problem with *oral* bio-identical estradiol is that it is rapidly broken down in the gut and liver before enough can be absorbed into the blood stream. Another concern about all *oral* estrogens is that they may increase liver production of clotting factors and raise levels of sex hormone binding globulin.
- Transdermal therapy regimens were developed in order to avoid some problems that can occur in association with the oral therapy, particularly the rapid breakdown of progesterone and estrogen by enzymes in the gut and liver before sufficient could be absorbed into the blood circulation. Transdermal hormone regimens are delivered from a small patch applied to the skin for continuous release of the hormone for up to a week.
- Hormone implants in the form of small pellets can be inserted into the fat of the abdomen or buttock for the slow release of estrogen or testosterone over a six to twelve month period. Unfortunately estrogen implants are no longer produced by the original pharmaceutical company but may be available from an Australian pharmaceutical source. Testosterone implants are still available and can be used.

- Troches or lozenges are used daily to deliver bio-identical hormones. The troche is prepared by compounding chemists in Australia according to a doctor's prescription. The troche is slowly absorbed through the mucous membrane of the mouth, but there are no studies to validate their efficacy or safety, and therefore are not approved by the Therapeutic Goods Administration (TGA).

CHAPTER 11

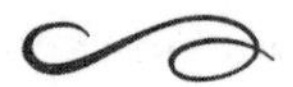

Adverse side-effects of HRT

There are positive and sometimes negative effects of any therapy. Medications of estrogen and progestogen are no exception, having side effects that can range from 'annoying' to 'harmful'. Annoying side effects can sometimes be tolerated and with adjustment of the treatment can be overcome. If a side-effect of a therapy is harmful then the therapy needs to be stopped, reassessed, changed and managed by the prescribing doctor. The most common known side effects of HRT are similar to those of the contraceptive pill and include breakthrough bleeding, painful breasts (mastalgia), skin changes, hair loss, excess growth of body hair, and weight gain.

Breakthrough bleeding

Breakthrough bleeding is abnormal bleeding from the uterus associated with a woman's sex hormone levels. For any woman using hormone therapy following her menopause, one of the most common complications causing anxiety is 'breakthrough' bleeding. The fear that the bleed is due to cancer of the uterus is the main concern, both for the woman who is bleeding and the doctor prescribing the therapy.

To help manage and deal with breakthrough bleeding, it is important to understand the physiological principles involved in producing the uterine bleed.

The majority of abnormal bleeds originate in the endometrium lining the uterus. Estradiol induces growth of the endometrium, so if estradiol is used by itself, the endometrium continues to proliferate until it is very thick, often developing cystic changes in the lush glandular tissue. The thick endometrium may outgrow its blood supply causing cells on the surface to die and expose the fragile blood vessels. The result of breakdown of this thick overgrowth of the endometrium (lining of the uterus) can be an excessively heavy bleed that sometimes requires blood transfusion and some form of surgical intervention. However this is now relatively rare as most therapies contain adequate amounts of a progestogen.

If the endometrium continues to be exposed to unopposed estrogen, the risk that the dividing cells in the endometrium will develop into endometrial cancer increases by about 1 per cent for every year that the estrogen is used.

The important principle for treating a woman who has a uterus, is to ensure that sufficient progestogen is added to the estrogen in order to prevent abnormal growth of the endometrium. To achieve adequate protection, it is usual to use a progestogen for at least two weeks in every month, but several variations to this advice are presently being advocated.

The majority of doctors suggest using a potent progestogen (like norethisterone, levonorgestrel, medroxyprogesterone acetate, drospirenone or dienogest) every day at a dosage that inhibits or prevents all endometrial cell division and therefore avoids the risk of abnormal endometrial cell proliferation. However, because there is continuing concern that some of the progestogens being used may have an adverse effect on other functions and organs, some doctors advocate using the progestogen for two weeks every one or two months or even only once in three months. These later regimens result in a withdrawal bleed within two to three days of stopping the progestogen, and because the endometrium is 'shed off', this method of prescribing progestogen reduces the risk of endometrial cancer.

Some healthcare advisers have promoted the concept of using the bio-identical progesterone as a transdermal cream or as a troche to inhibit endometrial cell division, but there is no reliable clinical evidence yet available to confirm that bio-identical progesterone administered in this form will be sufficient to control endometrial growth.

Using regular combined estrogen/progestogen therapy, the endometrium is occasionally so suppressed by the progestogen that growth through cell duplication never occurs, not even to replace cells which have undergone normal senescence (death through normal ageing). As a result, the blood vessels that normally provide nutrients to the growing endometrium are exposed, allowing a slight ooze of blood to take place through the very thin atrophic endometrial cell layer. Although this very slight, dark bleeding is relatively common in the first three months following initiation of therapy, it is rarely due to any significant lesion, but it does cause some concern until its cause is identified.

Investigation of breakthrough bleeding usually involves:

1. A gynaecological examination to confirm that a woman still has her uterus. If the uterus has been removed by hysterectomy, the bleeding could originate from some other part of the genital tract or even from the bladder, urethra or the lower bowel.
2. Examination of the vagina, cervix and uterus to ensure that there is no pathological lesion such as a growth or ulcer present in the parts of the genital tract that are not usually adversely affected by the administration of HRT.
3. Assessing the hormone therapy being used. Is estrogen being used alone or is it being used in combination with a progestogen?
4. Ultrasound assessment of the pelvis to determine whether the endometrium is thin (atrophic) or has evidence of hyperplasia, a polyp, a fibroid or a tumour.

Management of breakthrough bleeding

If no abnormality is detected by ultrasound, the regimen of HRT should be stopped for one week. This withdrawal of hormone support for the endometrium often results in a withdrawal bleed, like a normal menstrual 'period'.

If the ultrasound has confirmed that no abnormal pathological lesion is present inside the uterus then the bleed will cease soon after the HRT is stopped. The HRT can then be re-initiated without any concern, or the dose, or the estrogen/progestogen ratio can be modified if the hormone is thought to be the cause of the bleeding. If the ultrasound suggests an abnormality such as thick endometrium, or a polyp, or a sub-mucous fibroid or a cancer, then hysteroscopy and curettage should be performed.

If the ultrasound shows a thin endometrium (less than 5mm) the bleeding is almost certainly due to too much progestogen compared to the available estrogen. In this case, all that is required is a modification of the HRT regimen to decrease the progestogen or increase the estrogen until the appropriate regimen is achieved.

Mastalgia

Mastalgia is the term used to describe breast pain and it affects 70 per cent of women at some stage in their lives. Because breast tissue is part of the sexual anatomy of a woman's reproductive system, it is dependent on sex hormones for development and maintenance. Breasts are composed of millions of glands capable of producing secretions and milk. Each gland leads by a short duct to common ducts, which eventually join larger ducts before these ducts collect together behind the nipple. These glands and ducts are like bunches of grapes suspended in the fat of the breast. The breast is maintained in a full firm state while ever the glands, ducts and fat are capable of responding to estrogen and progesterone produced by the ovary. The breasts in a young woman remain well supported by strands of fibrous tissue embedded in the fat of each breast, but as a woman ages or the breasts become large and heavy, the fibrous strands stretch and the breasts sag.

The ducts and glands of the breast are supplied with nutrition and hormones by a complex network of arteries, veins, lymphatics and nerves, which run through and around each duct and gland. All the cells in the breast are hormone-sensitive, including the fat, the glands, the ducts and the breast support tissue.

When a woman passes the menopause and her production of estradiol and progesterone fails, the hormone responsive breast tissue begins to undergo atrophic (shrinking) changes. The ducts lose their elasticity and the glands shrink in size. The fibrous support strands lose strength as they stretch, allowing the breasts to sag under the weight of the fat in the breast, while benign fibrous tissue sometimes accumulates around glands to produce a rubbery mass of glands, ducts, and fibrous tissue called benign fibroadenosis (fibrocystic) change. Ducts in the fat become more obvious to palpation and to X-ray imaging in the atrophic breast.

When a woman with atrophic breast changes typical of the menopause is given HRT, the cells in the glands and ducts begin to regenerate and grow again. As this takes place, the nerves surrounding each gland are stretched, sometimes causing discomfort and even severe mastalgia. A woman who experiences breast discomfort can be advised that mastalgia caused by HRT will gradually settle over two to four weeks and that the pain is not an indication that something is wrong.

For women who find that mastalgia is intolerable, advice should be given to stop the therapy for one to two weeks to reduce the stimulating influence, or to try a less stimulating HRT regimen, such as tibolone (Livial) for three to six months, as it induces less breast discomfort than regular HRT.

Skin, hair growth and hair loss

Some women worry that regular HRT use may cause either loss of hair or excess growth of hair, in places not expected or wanted in a woman. Estrogen will not induce either loss or gain of hair but progestogens and testosterone may occasionally have a mild influence on the quality of hair. Estradiol improves the quality of the skin by inducing more production and deposition of collagen, giving the skin a thicker more supple quality compared with women deprived of estrogen. This improvement also applies to the skin in areas such as the vagina, while testosterone has a major growth stimulating effect on the cells in the clitoris and vulva as well as in the skin.

Following the menopause, and in the absence of estrogen, it is found that up to 15–20 per cent of the collagen in skin is depleted, leaving it thin, dry and fragile. It is easily traumatised by the simplest of knocks resulting in small bleeds (haematomas) under the surface.

Not only does the skin in a post-menopausal woman lose its ability to protect against trauma, but the hair growing from the skin becomes sparser and coarser while an older woman is often embarrassed by a few long, dark hairs on her face and chin. These dark hairs are not caused by hormones but are part of the ageing process.

Both males and females are born with the total number of hair follicles they will ever have. At birth, fine hair (lanugo) grows from each follicle and this fine hair remains for most of a female's life – seen in adults as a fine, downy, almost fluffy growth on the face and body. However, as a woman ages, the fine hair becomes darker and coarser. For a post-menopausal woman, the absence of estradiol and continual presence of low levels of androgens from the adrenal gland may increase the natural growth of fine hair.

In spite of these normal signs of ageing, the skin of some women may be affected by male hormones, which are produced either by the ovary or by the adrenal gland. Under the influence of androgen hormones, either prescribed by doctors or produced endogenously (within the body), the prolonged presence of androgens (testosterone or androstenedione) may increase the rate of growth of hair on the face, limbs or body.

Sometimes androgens (testosterone, androstenedione) cause so much growth of the surface cells of the skin that these surface cells, crowding together at the entrance to the follicle, obstruct the opening of the hair follicle that an acne-like pustule forms.

Weight gain

Everyone gains weight if they eat more food than they burn up (metabolise). Equally, burning up the total caloric intake in the ingested food results in loss of weight. However, there are many factors that are capable of interfering with this simple equation resulting in major difficulties for some people attempting to maintain an ideal body mass index (BMI). Both men and women inherit particular body shape and metabolic function from their parents, so these features cannot be changed. However, the outcome of every person's physical appearance can be modified by exercise, eating habits and personal interventions such as diet control, type of food, and type of physical activity.

Other hormones that also play a part in regulating body metabolism include thyroxin and progesterone. Progesterone is an inhibitor of the automatic contraction (peristaltic waves) of smooth muscle (found in the uterus, bladder, gut and gall bladder), resulting in a sensation of bloating and abdominal distention. In studies on HRT, it has been found that 80 per cent of women do not change weight over 12 months. Up to 10 per cent of women gain weight while 10 per cent lose weight while using HRT.

As a result of variation in the level of hormones influencing appetite, the desire for food varies from hour to hour and from day to day, so that no person ever requires or responds identically to the same level of a hormone as her neighbour, her sister or her friend. For some post-menopausal women, the use of regular HRT may disrupt the normal hormone sequence controlling appetite and metabolism, causing sudden changes in weight, exercise capability, body shape and fluid balance.

'Synthetic' progestogens are the sex hormones that are most likely to have an impact on weight and body shape. It is for this reason that some doctors promote the feasibility of using bio-identical progesterone, in combination with estradiol, to treat a post-menopausal woman. While weight control for some women becomes very difficult because of the complex interplay of the many different hormones involved in appetite, metabolism and weight loss, every woman using HRT should be aware that, for most, the sex hormones play only a peripheral role in the weight gain/loss equation.

Most adverse reactions of HRT can be easily solved once the underlying cause is identified and corrected.

Summary

- There are positive and sometimes negative effects of any therapy.
- A negative side effect of a therapy can range from 'annoying' to 'harmful' and these can be dealt with by adjusting the therapy or sometimes by stopping it altogether if it is causing harm.
- The most common known side-effects of HRT are similar to those of the contraceptive pill.
- These side effects include breakthrough bleeding, painful breasts, skin changes, hair loss, and excess growth of body hair and weight gain.
- Breakthrough bleeding is abnormal bleeding from the uterus in the presence of sex hormones.
- The most common cause of breakthrough bleeding is due to atrophy of the endometrium because of progestogen activity preventing normal cell regeneration.

- Insufficient progestogen allows overgrowth of the endometrium of the uterus sometimes causing excessive thickening of the lining.
- Progestogen in the right dosage is important in controlling the endometrium.
- Breakthrough bleeding must be investigated in order to determine its cause and to eliminate other causes for the bleeding.
- Mastalgia is a term that describes breast pain and it affects 70 per cent of women at some stage in their lives. Mastalgia develops because of hormonal stimulation of the breasts.
- While the ovaries produce estrogen and progesterone, the breasts can maintain their form, but as the ovaries begin to fail to produce their hormones during the perimenopause, the breasts also begin to fail to main their integrity.
- A woman who chooses to have HRT may initially experience mastalgia because the HRT stimulates her breast cells to regenerate. This should gradually settle over a period of two to four weeks.
- Adjusting the dosages of HRT to a less stimulating regimen may relieve mastalgia.
- The skin of a post-menopausal woman loses its ability to remain supple and firm, however estradiol improves the quality of skin, including the cells of the vagina and the clitoris.
- The skin of a post-menopausal woman can lose its ability to protect against trauma and she can easily sustain bleeding under the skin's surface.
- Occasionally the influence of androgens such as testosterone can cause an excess growth of the surface cells of the skin that they obstruct the surface cells of the hair follicles and result in acne-like pustules.
- There can be changes to the quality and quantity of a woman's hair. Estrogen does not induce either loss or gain of hair, but progestogens and testosterone may occasionally have a mild influence on the quality of a woman's hair. Any unwanted changes can be dealt with by adjusting her HRT.
- Weight control for some women becomes very difficult because of the complex interplay of the many different hormones involved in appetite, metabolism and weight loss, but a woman using HRT needs to be aware that for most, the sex hormones play only a very small role in weight gain or loss.

- 'Synthetic' progestogens are the sex hormones that have an impact on weight and body shape. It is for this reason that some doctors promote the feasibility of using bio-identical progesterone in combination with estradiol in order to treat a post-menopausal woman.
- Most adverse reactions of HRT can be easily identified and corrected with adjustment of a woman's HRT regimen.

CHAPTER 12

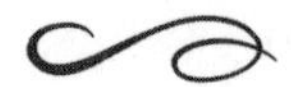

Other medical treatments for the menopause

Some women want or need to avoid the use of HRT but still want to prevent problems such as osteoporosis, cardiovascular adverse events such as heart attacks, stroke, thrombosis, embolus and cancers that are estrogen-dependent. To achieve this, lifestyle changes and a variety of therapies are promoted. One of these therapies is the group of selective estrogen receptor modulators (SERMs) and another is neurotransmitter modulators.

Specific estrogen receptor modulators (SERMs)

All cells that are dependent on estrogen for their function contain two different receptors, each one capable of initiating a different action within the cell. Each receptor requires a co-regulator that controls whether the action is to promote or inhibit the cell activity.

Selective Estrogen Receptor Modulators (SERMs) are designed medications that are capable of turning-on or turning-off a co-regulator for one of the two estradiol receptors within the nucleus of a cell. SERMs can activate the estrogen receptor and controls the cell activity by influencing the co-regulator. Sometimes it enhances co-regulator activity and sometimes it blocks co-regulator activity.

A characteristic that distinguishes SERMs is that their action is different in various tissues.

SERMs are a class of medications that are designed to act on a specific co-regulator of one or other of the estrogen receptors. A characteristic that distinguishes SERMs from estradiol is that their action is different in various tissues depending on the action of the co-regulator.

The choice of SERM depends on its pattern of action in various parts of the body. In circumstances where estrogen therapy is contraindicated, SERMs may be good replacements for HRT. For example, Raloxifene is used in the treatment of osteoporosis and may reduce the *risk* of breast cancer, while Tamoxifen is used to inhibit the action of estrogen on breast cancer cells in the *treatment* of breast cancer. In other words Tamoxifen blocks the action of estrogen on receptors in breast cancer cells.

Some cells either have predominantly α-estrogen receptors or β-estrogen receptors. A SERM is capable of creating different actions within the same cell or from different cells depending on the types of receptors within the cell.

These receptors activate the response within the nucleus of the cell but the receptors require co-regulators to dictate how that activity should be carried out.

Some co-regulators can activate *promotion* of cell division while others *prevent* cell division.

Breast and endometrial cells have predominantely Estradiol α-Receptor (α-ER), initiating growth and cell division within the breast, while bone and brain cells have mostly Estradiol β-Receptor (β-ER).

SERMs have been developed with the aim of promoting cell response for some characteristics of estrogen, at the same time preventing other estrogen responses.[103]

The first generation SERMs such as Clomiphene, Tamoxifen and Toremifene were developed to prevent osteoporosis and at the same time have preventive action on certain estrogen-dependent cells such as in the breast and brain and to have a stimulating effect on the uterus and endometrium. The endometrial stimulating function of these early SERMs was unacceptable for healthy women because of the increased risk of bleeding and uterine cancer, so they were abandoned as a means of treating women to reduce the risk of osteoporosis.

Second generation SERMs such as Raloxifene, were found to enhance and induce a beneficial action on bone with no increase in growth of cells in the uterus or the breast. Unfortunately there was no remission of flushes or sweats or improvement in lubrication or elasticity of the vaginal epithelium.

Among the newer SERMs being developed are those such as Bazedoxifene[104] – which in combination with an estrogen (Premarin) has resulted in remission of menopause symptoms, improvement in bone structure and has no adverse effect on the breast or uterus.

SERMs may be prescribed:

- To improve bone regeneration and reduce postmenopausal osteoporosis.
- To decrease breast cancer risk.

Various SERMs are listed and explained in Appendix 5.

Neurotransmitter modulators used for menopause

When a woman of menopausal age consults her doctor because of symptoms of stress, anxiety, mood swings, irritability, insomnia, inability to cope, sudden outbursts of anger, tears or fluctuating emotions, she is often diagnosed as being depressed or suffering from some psychiatric illness. Her busy doctor may make a diagnosis of depression and prescribe an anti-depressant. While this therapy may be necessary and anti-depressants may help a number of women who are suffering from a psychiatric illness, it may be the incorrect therapy and may even compound and accentuate the adverse symptoms caused by hormone deficiency.

Over many years, a number of women have noticed that the various non-hormone therapies they have been using have resulted in partial or complete remission of their menopausal symptoms. Scientifically constructed clinical studies have been conducted to confirm whether neurotransmitter modulators do have a beneficial effect on menopausal symptoms. It is the *interpretation of the results of these studies* that is sometimes misconstrued, sometimes misinterpreted and sometimes misrepresented by supporters of these therapies, so it is important to carefully review the reports in all such studies.

The use of a placebo alone will reduce menopausal symptoms in 50 per cent of women, so any therapy regimen must improve these symptoms by a statistically significant amount for it to be considered as valuable for management of the menopause.

Regimens that have received the most attention as potentially improving flushes and sweats are those that act on the neurotransmitters in the brain.

Neurotransmitters are chemicals produced in nerve cells. They are responsible for enabling messages to pass from one nerve cell to another.

Neurotransmitters fall into two main categories – they either excite or stimulate, or they inhibit or block.

A good example of a neurotransmitter is serotonin, which is regarded as the body's chemical of wellbeing. Serotonin is a very simple neurotransmitter that helps us to maintain our 'happy feelings' by regulating anger, aggression, body temperature, mood, sleep, sexuality and appetite. If the action of serotonin is disordered, then there may be an increase in aggressive and angry behaviour, clinical depression, obsessive-compulsive disorder, migraine, irritable bowel syndrome, tinnitus, fibromyalgia, bipolar disorder and anxiety disorders.

Excessive production of serotonin may cause an increase in hot flushes and sweats.

Over 50 different neurotransmitters have been identified and more are being detected.

Neurotransmitters currently being investigated as suitable for intervention therapies are:

- Amino acids such as glutamate, aspartate, aminoglutyric acid.
- Glycine mono-amines such as dopamine, nor-ethisterone, adrenaline, histamine and serotonin.
- Others such as acetycholine, adenosine, nitric acid and the endorphins.

Women who are deprived of the ovarian hormones often experience marked disturbance of their normal mental equilibrium. They may have memory loss, difficulty in solving even simple problems, disturbance of their emotions, have marked mood swings and may often act in a bizarre manner, completely at odds with their prior behaviour pattern. It is because of these manifestations of abnormal behaviour, that women are often treated with an anti-depressant. While these therapies may be important in management of a woman, it is important that her family physician take a careful history, not only of the symptoms disturbing her, but determine when the symptoms were first noticed or identified, what was the relationship with her periods, and were there any other symptoms suggesting a hormonal onset of the symptoms.

If there is a disorder of the action of a neurotransmitter then the use of a neurotransmitter modulator can restore the proper action of the neurotransmitter.

A modulator is something that regulates, adjusts, softens or tones down an action.

Anti-depressants modulate neurotransmitter activity in the brain.

There are many known neurotransmitter modulators. Chemical modulators that may block, reverse or enhance these different neurotransmitters are being invented. Because it is difficult to identify which nerve cells produce a particular range of neurotransmitters, the various modulators being developed are frequently investigated in trials on humans to identify what response will result from a particular drug. As a result, a number of unexpected consequences are often reported.

Some neurotransmitter modulators reduce hot flushes and vaso-motor symptoms, while other modulators simulate the neurotransmitter and may exacerbate menopausal symptoms. Some may induce abnormal and self-destructive actions in a person while others may produce erotic thoughts or increased sexual desire.

Some women on anti-depressants have improved considerably not only in their psychological and neurological health, but some also report a reduction in their hot flushes and sweats. It is because of this effect that a number of doctors are choosing to offer women who are experiencing flushes and sweats one of the anti-depressants as their first-line therapy. Anti-depressant treatment is usually suggested in order to avoid the perceived 'risk' associated with the use of regular HRT but some women who are given an anti-depressant will have vastly abnormal responses including drowsiness, hallucinations, and an increase in depression and abnormal behavioural responses such as maniacal activity or suicidal thoughts. Anti-depressants are not target specific but they affect all cells that produce a particular neurotransmitter for which it was designed.

The neurotransmitter modulators that have received the most attention as having a potential for improving hot flushes and sweats are Venlafaxine (Efexor), Desvenlafaxine (DVS), Escitalopram (Lexapro), Gabapentin (Neurontin), Catapres (Clonidine), Veralopride and Flibanserin. A description of the neurotransmitter inhibiters and enhancers that may potentially be useful for menopausal symptoms can be found in Appendix 6.

Summary

- SERMs are very beneficial for a post-menopausal woman who requires therapy to treat distressing symptoms of the menopause, but is unable to use regular estrogen.
- SERMs are synthesised chemicals that are capable of selectively activating or inhibiting one of the estrogen receptor co-regulators.
- SERMs have been designed to specifically target one or other of the estrogen receptors within cells
- The greatest value of SERMs is in reducing the **risk** of breast cancer at the same time as stimulating bone regeneration.
- Neurotransmitters are needed for healthy functioning of the brain.
- A neurotransmitter modulator such as an anti-depressant is a chemical that can restore the proper action of a neurotransmitter. Many women who have been prescribed a neurotransmitter modulator for symptoms of mood disturbance have reported that their menopausal vaso-dilator symptoms such as flushes and sweats have been relieved.
- Neurotransmitter modulators may help a menopausal woman who is experiencing problems with memory, mood swings and tearfulness,

irritability and depression but they do not protect a woman in the post-menopause against Alzheimer's dementia, cardiovascular disease or osteoporosis.

- During the peri-menopause a woman may feel depressed, teary, anxious and have mood changes and emotional outbursts. Some doctors may prescribe an anti-depressant (neurotransmitter modulator) for her when what might be of benefit for her is estrogen therapy.

CHAPTER 13

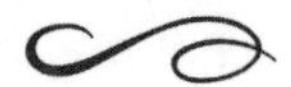

Complementary medicine and alternative therapies for menopause

Complementary and Alternative medicine (CAM) is regarded as any healing practice that does not fall within the realm of conventional or orthodox medicine. It is based on historical or cultural tradition, rather than on scientific evidence.

For a variety of reasons CAM therapies have been used by up to 75 per cent of the population to treat a variety of ills and diseases. In the United States, in the United Kingdom, in Australia, in Italy, and many other countries, surveys have been conducted to determine what Complementary and Alternative (CAM) therapies have been used, who has used them, the user age groups and for what reason. The most common CAMs being used are acupuncture, chiropractic, hypnotherapy, herbal medicine, osteopathy, homeopathy and over-the-counter preparations. Anecdotal responses suggest that about 90 per cent of users believe that the therapy has improved their symptoms but very few of the CAM therapies have ever been subjected to properly conducted placebo-controlled studies. Women are found to use CAM therapy almost twice as frequently as men and are more likely to buy over-the-counter therapy than men.

In 2002, a study conducted in the United States into the use of alternative therapy for menopausal women found that 76.1 per cent had used a CAM at some time in the previous twelve months. The most common reason for using an alternative therapy was for stress management (43 per cent). Over-the-counter therapy was sought by 37 per cent of users, a chiropractor was consulted by 31.6 per cent, massage was sought by 29 per cent, soy products by 23 per cent, acupuncture by 10.5 per cent, naturopathy or homeopathy by 9.5 per cent and herbal or Chinese medicine by 4.5 per cent. A CAM rather than orthodox therapy was sought by 22 per cent of women for treatment of hot flushes, sweats or insomnia.[105]

In an editorial of the *Medical Journal of Australia* it has been suggested that further research be conducted on various CAMs to determine whether they are effective or not, but no government or the CAM industry has been prepared to provide the huge financial investment necessary to determine whether any one of the many therapies, on offer to the population, is effective.[106] The only Level 1 studies that have been carried out have been conducted by medical scientists working in universities, but the size of, and length of time of such a study is always limited by the amount of money and time that is allowed for the study by the university administration.

Either a therapy works or it doesn't. If it doesn't work it must be considered as nothing more than a placebo. Promotion of a useless product as a cure of symptoms or even as a relief of symptoms denies the consumer access to, or the right, to a proper diagnosis.

It was found in a telephone survey in the United Kingdom that 44 per cent of women were using an alternative therapy regimen for menopausal symptoms with the most popular being Evening Primrose Oil (54 per cent), followed by vitamins (42 per cent), St John's Wort (18 per cent), and extracts of red clover and soy at 10 per cent each, also being consumed.[107]

Universally, it has been found that a women decides to use various extracts of herbal or non-traditional therapy regimens following recommendations from friends, their hairdresser, from pharmacists or based on advertisements in newspapers or women's magazines. In very few instances in the various surveys were alternative therapies recommended by the medical profession.

Why do so many women use alternative therapies that have not been endorsed by qualified health professionals?

Part of the answer to this dilemma lies with the fact that some members of the health professions dismiss a woman's symptoms as being irrelevant and not requiring treatment. Allied with the universal scepticism regarding the motives of the medical profession and the pharmaceutical industry, women have become disenchanted. Exposure of some false claims by the pharmaceutical industry for various preparations, or for the failure of other companies to provide all the information regarding trials on drugs that are being developed, has led to increasing scepticism of statements regarding therapy for the menopause. Many members of the medical profession have been criticised for associating themselves with these claims by the pharmaceutical companies.

Exposure of false claims has often resulted in rejection of the belief that hormones are a benefit for post-menopausal women. Allied to this healthy scepticism has been the influence of the media, which promotes negative or opposing research findings or which quotes the varied opinions held by health professionals who promote different or controversial points of view. The media has quite rightly encouraged discussion of controversial issues by presenting information regarding such topics, but in order to provoke interest and discussion with readers, some correspondents have presented a distorted conclusion regarding the subject, and then encourage comment from 'experts' in order to stimulate further discussion. This reporting device has been used with effect (particularly about breast cancer) and has often led to extreme statements being made when personal or fixed opinions are challenged.

However, one cannot blame the media alone for the poor image of HRT. The medical profession is also at fault for not adequately educating the public, the media and other health professionals regarding the benefits and adverse effects of hormone therapy.

The final reason that women seek alternative therapies lies with the promoters of alternative therapies. There is very little control or legislation preventing any person claiming that a particular product may be used for a specific problem. As a consequence, some 'health shop' proprietors, some pharmaceutical companies, some independent practitioners and even some dispensing pharmacists have claimed that a particular product or extract is helpful for menopausal women, without conducting any scientific research, or for providing proof of efficacy or of safety of a product.

The major dilemma for patients when choosing to use an alternative therapy for menopausal symptoms is in distinguishing 'good oil' which is beneficial, from 'snake oil' which is not.

Jennifer's story

Around the age of 48, pre-menopause hit. I had the usual problems of hot flushes and night sweats and the sleepless nights affected me badly. Fortunately after a bit of trial and error, my GP prescribed a contraceptive pill for me. All my symptoms went and all was well for a few years until my periods stopped and my GP decided that I was definitely in menopause and that it would be safe to now stop taking the pill. My GP explained that research showed that there was an increased health risk if I continued taking hormones.

When I stopped taking the pill, all my symptoms returned. So my doctor prescribed many alternatives, all with very low doses of hormones for 'safety' reasons. Each new prescription took about three to five weeks to take effect, which meant that months passed and I was suffering terribly. I started consulting other general practitioners and was getting the same cautious advice, the same prescriptions, but no relief!

After about nine months of misery, I decided to visit a specialist who confirmed that the evidence from large studies in America was alarmist. More careful analysis showed that for younger, healthier females just entering menopause, estrogen balanced with progestin, overall, was beneficial for women. At long last I received a prescription with enough hormones to stop the terrible problems I was having.

My journey wasn't quite finished though! I moved to a different area, where I visited a different GP who specialised in 'holistic medicine', and who convinced me to start on natural hormones called bio-identical hormones where the amounts could be individually tailored to my needs by a compounding pharmacy. My symptoms returned and worsened. I started to get dizzy spells and mental confusion and vagueness. I visited another GP, recommended by the compounding pharmacy.

This GP recommended a liver-cleansing diet as my body was clearly not absorbing my supplemental hormones. She also recommended additional saliva tests, liver tests and herbal supplements organised through her practice. My alarm bells were ringing. More of my research revealed to me that the bio-identical hormone I was prescribed could not alleviate my symptoms but when I mentioned this to the GP she responded that it would be 'dangerous for my health to continue on strong, synthetic formulations! Weak and natural was safer for me'. *It was also ineffective!*

I've learnt my lesson. Stick to what is sound science and be suspicious of alternatives, even natural ones! I now find relief with HRT.

Proof of efficacy

The evidence to support a claim for a benefit of any therapy regimen should be impeccable, the results should be relevant to the disease or problem being treated, and the studies must include sufficient numbers of women to allow a firm conclusion to be drawn as to the statistical validity of the claims.

It is of little relevance to attempt to substantiate a claim for a therapy by saying it has been used for hundreds of years and therefore it must be okay, or of saying that a friend had tried a product and it had 'cured' her of her ailment, or to say that because a reputable therapy such as acupuncture relieves pain, it will have a beneficial effect on post-menopausal symptoms. There does need to be adequate research carried out to validate the claim.

To date the proponents or promoters of many alternative therapies have failed to produce any material evidence to substantiate the many claims that a particular product will achieve a benefit and instead they have relied on anecdotal accounts and Level 3 research findings. This is clearly unsatisfactory for patients and doctors who are trying to decide on the merits of a particular regimen of therapy. The benefits of any alternative therapy must be identified through properly conducted research using prospective, double-blind, placebo-controlled trials.

Following is a review of just some of these products and the claims and justification being made for their use.

Vitamins

Vitamins have been used widely by women in the belief that, if a certain amount of a particular vitamin is essential for health, taking twice or more times the base amount will provide two or three times as much benefit.

Unfortunately consuming larger amounts of some vitamins does not convey any advantage. In fact, consuming larger quantities of vitamins may even be counterproductive – excessive amounts of Vitamin B may lead to neurological damage while Vitamin A may induce adverse effects in the liver.

However, at least one vitamin is thought to convey an advantage for a woman if consumed in amounts above the normal range found in the average population. Vitamin C is a powerful antioxidant and because of this action is believed to reduce the risk of cardiovascular disease and even some cancers.

In spite of multi-vitamins being readily available in most pharmacies and health food shops an informed health care provider needs to be responsible for supervising the augmentation of a diet with vitamin supplements.

The famous Women's Health Initiative (WHI) Study[108] recruited almost 162,000 women, of whom half were given added vitamins for eight years. There was no significant difference in the incidence of cancer, cardiovascular disease or other major illnesses when those taking the added vitamins were compared to the group of women who were not given any added vitamins.

The only known exception to the conclusion that there is no advantage in adding vitamins to a well-balanced diet, is in regard to the addition of Vitamin D to the diet to enhance uptake of calcium and improve bone mineral density. There is some evidence that added Vitamin D may reduce the incidence of cancer and heart attacks, and several studies have suggested that Vitamin D in appropriate dosage does have a beneficial effect on all cells, apart from those involved in calcium metabolism.

Soy products

Some of the popular alternative therapies include extracts of the soy plant. This plant product gained major publicity following release of reports that Japanese women experienced fewer vaso-motor symptoms and developed less breast cancer than similar aged women in the United States. In attempting to identify the causes for these differences, the consumption of animal fats by Americans and the widespread use of soy products by Japanese were targeted as potential associated factors.

Soy contains a large concentration of isoflavones, and it was this group of compounds that was thought to alleviate menopause symptoms as well as to reduce the risk of breast cancer. However, although there is some laboratory data to suggest that some isoflavones may increase maturation and differentiation of breast cells, there is very little long-term clinical or epidemiological data available to support the hypothesis that soy products stop hot flushes, reduce osteoporosis, dementia, heart attacks or reduce the risk of breast cancer.

Prospective, randomised, double-blind research studies reviewing the effect of soy products on distressing hot flushes and sweats have failed to produce convincing evidence that soy has a comprehensive beneficial effect on these vaso-motor symptoms. The available evidence suggests that the phyto-estrogens in soy products do have a slight affinity for the estrogen receptors in human females but any reduction in hot flushes has occurred only among women who have mild or occasional symptoms.

Of some significance for women accustomed to consuming a Western diet is the fact that the amount of soy products thought necessary to provide protection from abnormal change is more than most women are willing to consume on a daily basis for long periods of time. Phyto-estrogen products, derived from soy are sold by manufacturers who advertise and promote them as 'natural' products.

There is no known adverse effect from using products derived from soy but the benefits are of a dubious value, and there are no long-term studies that support the concept that soy products lessen the risk of osteopaenia or cardiovascular disease.

However, because of the possibility that over time, women using soy products may gain an overall benefit, those who have begun such a therapy regimen may be encouraged to continue to use soy products, even though it is difficult to endorse them as a primary treatment of menopause symptoms.

Red clover extract (*Promensil*)

Because red clover also contains a large amount of isoflavones, (genestein, diadzein), an extract of red clover (Promensil) was marketed with the belief that these phyto-oestrogens would not only be beneficial for post-menopausal symptoms, but would also avoid any adverse effects which are currently associated with the use of orthodox hormone therapy.

Many studies have now been conducted into the efficacy of Promensil. Unfortunately, not only did Promensil not relieve vaso-motor symptoms any better than the placebo, but there have been no studies indicating that it had a beneficial effect on osteoporotic bone fractures, heart attacks or on the risk of dementia, nor were there any safety studies available to prove it did not exert an adverse effect if taken long term.

Black cohosh (*Remifemin*)

Black cohosh is a plant that contains triterpene glycosides. It was used extensively by North American Indians at the time of colonisation to treat various illnesses, including fevers, and eventually the plant and its extracts found its way back to the 'old world' where healthcare therapists cultivated the plant for use by apothecaries. In Germany, an industry has recently grown up devoted to the extraction of, and use of, the product obtained from the black cohosh plant. It is sold in Australia as Remifemin. The glycoside extracts of the black cohosh are thought to have a weak estrogenic activity and, as such, Remifemin has been promoted as an alternative to estrogen to treat menopausal symptoms. Because of the extensive promotion of Remifemin both in the lay press and medical journals it has become the most commonly used CAM for treating menopausal symptoms.

Studies have confirmed that it has a mild influence on reducing flushes, but it appears to have no apparent positive effect on vaginal epithelium, on skin or bone and no effect on the breast. In several studies, Remifemin has proven to be better than a placebo in controlling vaso-motor symptoms, but the positive effects are not universal and women generally have been disappointed after long-term use, as other adverse changes of hormone deficiency continue to occur.

A randomised, placebo-controlled trial comparing the effectiveness of black cohosh, red clover extract, estradiol and a placebo, resulted in the remission of flushes and sweats after one year for each of these treatments, but red clover extract failed to be as effective as the placebo, and the black cohosh was even less effective as the following results of the trial demonstrate.

Table 5:

FLUSHES AND SWEATS (improvement after one year)[109]	
BLACK COHOSH	34 per cent
RED CLOVER EXTRACT	57 per cent
PLACEBO	63 per cent
ESTRADIOL	94 per cent

Preparations of black cohosh have been associated with serious hepatic reactions and caution has been expressed by Adverse Drug Reaction Committees.[110] Forty-nine cases of massive necrosis of the liver have been reported following the use of extracts of black cohosh, some occurring within a few months of starting treatment.[111]

Evening primrose oil

For over twenty years, evening primrose oil has been promoted as having extraordinary powers in improving wellbeing in humans. However, it is worth noting the pedigree and constituents of evening primrose oil. Common farm crops such as sunflower, Canola, olives and other plants including the evening primrose flower can be crushed to extract oils which contain a group of fatty acids such as gamolenic acid and other omega-6 fatty acids. These fatty acids are the precursors for a group of products (arachidonic acids), which can be further metabolised to some of the essential signalling molecules in the human female. Because arachidonic acid is intimately involved, as a precursor, in developing these specific messengers for communicating specific functions in women, the promoters of the use of evening primrose oil have suggested that this product is capable of improving the metabolic activity associated with a number of dysfunctions ranging from mastalgia through to painful periods, PMT and menopausal symptoms.

The evening primrose flower contains the same oils and produces a similar selection of omega fatty acids such as linolenic acid and gamma-linoleic acid as do the domestic margarines. The best that can be said about evening primrose oil is that it is an expensive plant oil, which does no harm, but which has never been shown to have any more medicinal effect than commercial margarine. In a variety of scientific studies involving double-blind, prospective, placebo-controlled trials, it has never been shown to have any beneficial effect for women suffering from menopausal problems, but it is often prescribed for women when there is no other effective treatment option.

Traditional Chinese herbal medicines

Examples of traditional Chinese herbal medicine include ginseng and dong quai.

These are popular Chinese herbal remedies that have been prescribed over many years for many symptoms including pre-menstrual syndrome, menopausal flushes, loss of libido and also for the promotion of wellbeing. Unfortunately, there is very little scientific evidence that they convey any clinical benefit. In fact, the only large placebo-controlled trial comparing ginseng with a placebo showed that the placebo was equally as effective as ginseng at controlling flushes. There have been no long-term studies to show that either dong quai or ginseng is effective or safe or harmful.

Some 'natural remedies' from Asian sources have been found to contain carcinogens, mutagens, neurotoxins and substances which can cause organ damage as well as some being contaminated with heavy metals and living organisms causing harm to the body and even death. Until the marketers of traditional Chinese medicines are prepared to subject their product to a properly conducted scientific study, funded by those who make substantial sums of money from sale of these products, the use of them is questionable.[112]

Progesterone cream

During the latter part of the 20th century, progesterone cream alone, without the addition of estradiol, was vigorously promoted by Dr John Lee, a family physician in California, as a therapy regimen to not only control hot flushes, but to prevent osteoporosis and other deleterious effects of the menopause.

While most clinicians are aware that the use of natural progesterone, in conjunction with appropriate amounts of estradiol, would be the preferred form of HRT to protect the endometrium from developing cancer, there is no credible evidence from scientific studies, that progesterone alone, administered as a cream, is capable of inhibiting hot flushes or of preventing osteoporosis. There is also considerable doubt that transdermal progesterone can be absorbed in sufficient amounts to inhibit endometrial cell proliferation. However, at least one study from France suggests that a transdermal cream, combining both estradiol and a progesterone, reduces menopausal symptoms without inducing an increase in vaginal bleeding, or increasing the risk of breast or uterine cancer.

Estradiol is active on cells in units of function measured in picomoles/L while progesterone is required in nanomoles/L quantities in order to be effective (1 nanomole is equivalent to 1000 picomoles). Unfortunately the amount of progesterone absorbed through the skin is similar in amount to that which is absorbed when estradiol is applied and, at this level, which is much less than is normally produced by the ovary, is insufficient to inhibit division and growth of endometrial cells.

Studies that have been conducted, suggest that progesterone in transdermal cream is not absorbed in sufficient amounts to have any major biological effect. Several well-conducted, prospective, double-blind, placebo-controlled trials have shown a slight increase in circulating levels of progesterone, when applying progesterone cream, but none of these studies have shown any effect on vaso-motor symptoms, mood, sexual feelings, vaginal tissue, bones or blood vessels.[113]

Until there is clear evidence that a progesterone cream is capable of delivering sufficient progesterone into the circulation to have an effect on vaso-vagal symptoms, to protect the endometrium, or to inhibit bone loss, then the advocacy and sale of transdermal progesterone cream, applied without estradiol, for treatment of the menopause, is unethical and irresponsible.

Administered in a transdermal cream, there is no credible evidence that progesterone reduces the risk of breast or endometrial cancer, or prevents osteoporosis or heart attacks and it certainly does not reduce flushes, sweats and insomnia, nor does it have a beneficial effect on a dry vagina.

Wild yam cream

Mexican wild yam contains a substance called diosgenin, which is the substrate capable of being converted in a laboratory by a complex sequence of enzymatic reactions to bio-identical progesterone. However, Mexican wild yam (and diosgenin by itself) has no effect on menopausal symptoms or on hormone-deficiency problems when used in its *natural* form. Humans do not have the necessary enzymes in their body that can convert diosgenin to progesterone. Therefore the use of creams containing Mexican wild yam have no impact on the menopause or on menopausal symptoms and the promotion of this product for treatment of menopausal symptoms could be unethical and possibly harmful. Women using these products gain no protection from any of the effects of hormonal deficiency. Instead, potentially life-threatening changes may develop which could have been prevented if appropriate therapy had been instituted instead of relying on wild yam cream. Wild yam creams are examples of snake oil – doing no good and potentially contributing to the long-term deterioration of post-menopausal women who use this therapy.

DHEAS (dehydroepiandrosterone sulphate)

Dehydroepiandrosterone sulphate (DHEAS) is a steroid product of the cortex of the adrenal gland. It is excreted in relatively large amounts in young people. DHEAS can be converted by enzymes to either dehydroepiandrosterone (DHEA) or to androstenediol (ADIOL). Both DHEA and ADIOL have been shown to induce growth of breast cells in culture.

The amount of naturally produced DHEA in the human body declines steadily from the age of 25 years and therefore has often been described as a 'youth hormone'. As a consequence, there has been an increasing advocacy to add DHEAS, DHEA or ADIOL to the group of hormones to maintain health and youth, particularly in post-menopausal women.

DHEAS is derived from the cholesterol molecule by enzymes in the adrenal gland, and is then further metabolised to androstenedione, testosterone or to estradiol by enzymes in various cells in the body. Unfortunately, DHEA does not have a direct action on cells in the same way that hormones do. No human protein receptors to which DHEA could attach, or induce a response within a cell, have been identified. For that reason DHEA is not to be regarded as a messenger hormone, however it can be converted by enzymes into either estradiol or testosterone, and therefore it can be regarded as a precursor of the normal sex hormones.

It is likely that any clinical response identified in women or animals is due to conversion of DHEA into estradiol or testosterone. Although DHEA has been promoted as a 'youth pill' conveying an extension of the joys of youth and prolonging life, there is no scientific evidence in humans to support such a claim. It has also been prescribed and sold as an alternative to standard hormone therapy with claims of an improvement in bone and the cardiovascular system, and an elevation in moods and wellbeing. The articles supporting these claims have been mostly of an anecdotal nature (Level 3 studies) or have been studies carried out on animals. It is likely that any improvement is the result of enzymatic conversion of DHEA into either estradiol or testosterone.

There have been no well-conducted scientific, prospective, double-blind placebo-controlled trials, nor credible clinical studies to support the claim that DHEA conveys any advantage to post-menopausal women that is not achieved by conventional HRT. Some recent reports have suggested that it may act as an anti-depressant, but the evidence is unconvincing and the improvement may merely reflect the action of estradiol and testosterone.

DHEA is not a messenger hormone in its own right. For it to be converted into an active hormone it requires many changes by enzymes in body cells before it achieves any positive action. It is a precursor to estradiol or testosterone.

Over-the-counter products

Many women entering pharmacies and health food shops are confronted with a range of products that have been produced by manufacturing companies for women who wish to reduce symptoms of the menopause but fear using regular therapy. These products have rarely been subjected to any credible research regarding efficacy or safety. Regulatory laws have been drafted to control the production and sale of a number of questionable products, while the Therapeutic Goods Administration (TGA) has not supported any claims that there is a benefit for symptoms of the menopause by the use of these products.

At present there is no legislation to force manufacturers of over-the-counter (OTC) products to warn a woman that there is no scientific evidence that the product being promoted may have any benefit. However labelling such as that of the TGA is available and is described in Appendix 1.

The manufacturers of OTC therapies have not conducted Level 1 trials that can establish the benefits or adverse or harmful effects of their product.

Women who use OTC products may obtain a beneficial response (the halo effect) similar to the response to a placebo (50 per cent improvement in flushes), but will not gain any advantage from a reduction in insomnia, a dry vagina with painful intercourse, osteoporosis, heart disease or dementia.

The use of, and reliance on, unproven therapies may actually be detrimental for women who have depended on OTC products to relieve symptoms. While there may be remission of flushes, OTC products have not been proven to prevent adverse physical changes. Prolonging their use allows continuing and sometimes irreversible deterioration of important organs and body tissue.

Summary

- The use of Complementary and Alternative (CAM) therapies to treat menopausal symptoms is widespread with up to 50 per cent of women using an alternative treatment for a period of time.
- There are anecdotal reports of partial or occasional remission of distressing flushes and sweats when any of the alternative therapies are employed, but there has never been any scientific evidence that they provide protection to the uterus, the breasts, the vagina, bones, arteries, heart, or brain cells.
- Many over-the-counter products contain a mixture from between two and up to twenty different products, all claimed without proof to provide an advantage for women using them during the menopause.
- Research into the efficacy of CAMs would identify the products that are effective and the products that are not.
- CAMs are not proven through controlled trials, so their continued use may delay a proper clinical examination and the introduction of an appropriate therapy regimen for each woman.
- Every woman deserves a consultation with a doctor who has expertise in managing the symptoms of the menopause. This consultation entails a pathology assessment of blood hormone levels, cholesterol levels and glucose levels; a full gynaecological examination including blood pressure and breast examination; a Pap smear; a mammogram and a bone density study.

- With information gained from these tests, a woman's test results need to be discussed with her, so that she can make her own choice about the therapy that best suits her as an individual.
- Hormone replacement therapy is not a 'one size fits all' approach. Each woman needs to be prescribed her own program according to her needs with regular routine follow-up assessments.
- Complementary and alternative therapies do not rely on proper assessment of the screening process and therefore deny a woman her 'full routine (annual) medical check-up'.
- The lack of comprehensive information about alternative and complementary therapies, may indicate that they are not suitable for many women seeking relief from their estrogen-deficiency symptoms.
- There is no evidence that CAMs protect a woman in her post-menopausal years from the risks of osteoporosis, heart disease, cancer and Alzheimer's dementia.

CHAPTER 14

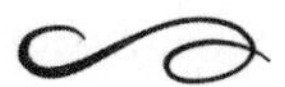

HRT following breast cancer, endometriosis or fibroids

A woman who has developed a debilitating condition such as endometriosis, or who has developed a fibroid (causing bleeding, pressure or pain), or has been treated for breast cancer, may be advised by her doctor to avoid the use of HRT. This advice is usually given because of the risk that hormone therapy will have a detrimental effect on the long-term outcome of her disease.

However, for a woman who experiences the distressing symptoms of menopause with some restriction on the use of hormone therapy to relieve those symptoms or to obtain relief from the mood swings and fluctuating emotions, life can become intolerable – even considered by some women as not worth living any longer! Some women have considered suicide following treatment for breast cancer when faced with the thought of years of misery without relief from the depressive effect of estrogen deficiency.

Many women, given a choice of either continuing to experience distressing menopausal symptoms without hormone therapy, or alternatively, using hormones with a possible regrowth of their cancer, choose to have immediate relief following estradiol therapy rather than continue to suffer from flushes, sweats or psychological or emotional distress.

The question arises in every case 'will the use of estrogen therapy have an adverse effect on the disease?' While there is no question that estrogen may make some breast cancers grow more rapidly, or to cause endometriosis to become active or continue the growth pattern of some fibroids, not all women reject estrogen following diagnosis and treatment of these diseases.

HRT after breast cancer

Anomalies that frequently occur when advice is offered regarding the use of hormone therapy following breast cancer are illustrated in the following stories and clinical details of three women.

A mother of two children was 39 when she was diagnosed with a right breast cancer in 1988. She had a mastectomy with removal of glands, followed by radiotherapy and chemotherapy. Every one of her 19 lymph nodes was involved in metastatic cancer and she was given a gloomy prognosis.

Soon after she had completed her chemotherapy, she ceased to menstruate and began to experience overwhelming flushes, sweats, insomnia and marked mood swings with depression. In turn, she was prescribed Clonidine, then an anti-depressant and finally Provera in a high dose, but her symptoms persisted. Her despair at the change in her life was so marked and miserable that she contemplated suicide rather than live her life as it was. She had asked her oncologist if she could use HRT, but both he and her surgeon refused to prescribe any therapy containing estrogen.

Finally, she was referred for a second medical opinion. This opinion concurred with her oncologist's view that estrogen could increase the spread of her cancer, but she felt that unless something was done to reduce her distressing symptoms, she might as well die anyway. After discussion, it was agreed that she could begin standard hormone therapy. Her symptoms, depression and mood swings improved immediately and she has remained on regular HRT ever since. Twenty-three years after her diagnosis and treatment of stage III breast cancer, she returns every year for a routine check-up. She is still concerned she may have a recurrence of her cancer but is otherwise very well. She works as a secretary, and she is still on estradiol and a progestin. At 62 years of age she has no menopausal symptoms and she leads a happy, physical, mental and sexually active life.

The story of the second woman is very different. She worked for a pharmaceutical company, was a heavy smoker, and was personally interested in a religious group that promoted natural therapy and prayer. Every few years she attended for a Pap smear and breast examination but she was not interested in any advice regarding medication for her own health even though she was responsible for promoting medications for her company. In 1983, at the age of 45 years, she developed a lump in her left breast that was possibly a cancer. A mammogram confirmed that there were signs suggesting a malignancy but instead of consulting a surgeon as recommended she decided to seek the advice of her religious leader who was also a naturopath. Four years later, she sought gynaecological advice regarding overwhelming flushes and insomnia. She had been post-menopausal for two years and in spite of using a potpourri of herbal therapy, prayers and meditation from her religious leader, she was unable to obtain relief. She had not received any therapy for the breast lesion and now had secondary malignant growths in her liver as well as in her brain. She realised that she was going to die from her cancer but wanted some relief from her hot flushes and insomnia. She commenced hormone therapy in the form of estrogen alone and had complete relief from her menopausal symptoms until she died five months later.

The third story of a woman, a doctor, who had HRT following breast cancer is best described in her own words:

> *I had a diagnosis of a grade 1 breast cancer in October 2005 (aged 45 years). I had a lumpectomy, followed by further clearance of lymph nodes, as the sentinel node had micro-metastasis. I then had radiotherapy and was put onto Tamoxifen, as the tumour was very oestrogen (and progesterone) receptor positive.*
>
> *Well, the Tamoxifen was terrible! I took it for 9 months – feeling very miserable and suicidal for the last 4 months (totally unlike me – always a cup half full to overflowing). I stopped feeling like a woman. Stopped feeling like me at all!*
>
> *Finally, I took myself off the Tamoxifen and started to feel better within days. My menstrual cycles re-established themselves and I even began to ovulate again.*
>
> *Then from 2008, I started to get menopausal symptoms, reminiscent of those experienced when on Tamoxifen.*
>
> *In April 2009, I was at a conference where breast cancer was discussed and following discussion, I decided to try HRT. I have had a progestogen IUD fitted and have begun on a transdermal oestrogen gel.*
>
> *I look and feel great – just look at my web page (and photo). I look younger and better than I did in 2000, exercise for 25 minutes every morning and feel like I am getting into my stride again. I have never had so much energy for life/sex/work. I feel like my old self again and my husband is delighted.*

These three women and their stories illustrate that there is never a situation where a woman who has had breast cancer should be precluded from being offered a form of hormone therapy if her symptoms are such that life without estrogen is intolerable.

Estrogen will make malignant cells with a receptor for estrogen grow more vigorously – but if there are no viable cancer cells left after appropriate surgery, radiotherapy and/or chemotherapy, then estrogen is unlikely to increase the risk of recurrence or death. The critical decision will depend on the probability of the cancer having been eliminated.

When considering the potential risk of spread, recurrence of the tumour and the woman's survival following a diagnosis of breast cancer, it is usual to evaluate the risks by using three criteria – the stage of the cancer, the grade of the cancer, and the hormone receptor status of the cancer.

The stage of the tumour refers to the extent of invasion of surrounding tissue by the cancer at the time of diagnosis. Traditionally a cancer is allocated to one of five stages in order to indicate how far the tumour has progressed in its invasion of the body. Breast cancer that has not invaded through the basement membrane into surrounding tissue is called cancer in-situ (stage 0). Adequate treatment cures over 95 per cent of cancer in-situ, while stage 1 (early invasion into breast tissue) is cured in over 80 per cent of women. When an invasive cancer has reached less than five glands in the axilla under the arm (stage 2) the cure rate drops to about 70 per cent while stage 3 (more than five glands involved) has a cure rate of closer to 50 per cent. Stage 4 cancers have already spread to other parts of the body, so a cure is very much less likely.

The grade of cancer is assessed according to how aggressive the cells appear to be. There are three grades of cancer and a pathologist interprets this grading.

The receptor status is the third criterion for assessment of a cancer and it identifies the potential response of the cells to hormones. This response depends on the presence or absence of estrogen or progesterone protein receptors in the cancer cells and is determined by a biopsy and special pathological analysis of the proteins in the cell.

Because of the excellent results following early detection, there has been a major emphasis on screening all 'at-risk' women to identify breast cancer while it can be cured. However, a debate is now taking place as to whether women diagnosed with cancer in-situ are actually at risk at all. There is evidence from long-term biopsy-controlled studies that at least 50 per cent of breast cancer in-situ never invades other tissue, never progresses and that some may even undergo spontaneous remission.[114]

Notwithstanding the debate over management of cancer in-situ, when an early stage cancer has been appropriately treated and potentially cured, the use of hormone therapy following a diagnosis of cancer does not cause a new cancer to develop, and when administered in a careful and considered regimen, hormone therapy is capable of enhancing quality of life without increasing mortality.

Several large studies, involving hormone therapy following breast cancer, have not demonstrated an increase in recurrence or death. In 1992 a group of 224 women, of whom 77 per cent were post-menopausal and who had been treated for breast cancer, were reviewed. Over three-quarters of the women believed they needed hormone therapy to treat their menopause symptoms, or to prevent heart disease and osteoporosis, and 60 per cent of them were prepared to take estrogen therapy under medical supervision.[115]

In 1998 in Australia, 1472 women with a history of breast cancer were reviewed. A total of 167 (11.3 per cent) in this study had used hormone therapy because of flushes and sweats following treatment for breast cancer. This review found that the risk of recurrence or development of a new cancer was not increased by the use of estrogen and it was concluded that the use of HRT following breast cancer was not contra-indicated among those who had a need for such therapy.[116] Other studies have also confirmed that women who have used HRT after breast cancer have not had an increased risk of recurrence or death.[117]

In a study published in 2001 by O'Meara in the United States, 2755 women with invasive breast cancer were identified. Of these women, 174 (6.32 per cent) had used HRT following their treatment for breast cancer. Relative risks of recurrence and death were estimated. The rate of breast cancer recurrence among women who used HRT after breast cancer was 17/1000 compared to 30/1000 women who did not use hormone therapy. Death due to breast cancer was 5/1000 in those using HRT compared to 15/1000 among women who avoided estrogen therapy. The conclusion was made that the risk of recurrence or death was lower among women using hormone therapy than among those who were not.[118]

From both individual accounts and cohort studies it would appear that HRT given to a woman who has been treated for breast cancer does not increase the risk of recurrence or death. However it is important to realise that the majority of women who elected to use an estrogen-based therapy after breast cancer had Stage 0, Stage 1 or Stage 2 breast cancer. The complete cure of these cancers is high and therefore the risk of recurrence and death is low.

Hormone therapy is not recommended for a woman who has had breast cancer, but if her symptoms of estrogen deficiency are so distressing that they adversely affect the capacity of a woman to enjoy life, then she can be advised that evidence suggests that women who have been treated for early stage cancer have no increased risk of recurrence or death following the use of HRT.

Young women who have developed breast cancer before their menopause are treated with surgical removal of the tumour, radiotherapy and frequently a form of chemotherapy. While it is acknowledged that estrogen may have an adverse effect on breast cancer, very few of these young women are advised to have their ovaries removed to reduce the risk. In fact, a number of women with breast cancer have become pregnant after their cancer has been treated and results from studies have suggested there is no greater risk of recurrence or death than among women who decide to avoid pregnancy.[119]

HRT and endometriosis

Endometriosis is a disease in which the mucous glands that normally line the cavity of the uterus have grown outside the uterus. These endometriotic deposits respond and grow under the influence of estrogen, often forming cysts and deposits of blood on the lining of the pelvic organs (peritoneum). As a result of the irritant effects of blood in the pelvis, women suffering from endometriosis frequently develop adhesions (the sticking together of organs such as the bowel, uterus and ovaries due to an inflammatory reaction). They have painful 'periods', pain during sexual intercourse; sub-fertility and bowel and bladder irritation. Following surgery to remove affected tissue, removal of ovaries, or when reaching their natural menopause, women with a history of endometriosis are often advised to avoid the use of estrogen as it may induce growth of endometriotic deposits again.

However, women with endometriosis can take estrogen to relieve their symptoms if the estrogen is accompanied by the administration of progestogen in a dose sufficient to inhibit the growth of the endometriotic deposits. A suitable regimen may include estradiol with a potent progestogen such as nor-ethisterone, levonorgestrel or dienogest.

HRT and fibroids (fibromyoma)

Fibroids grow from cells in the wall of arteries supplying the uterus. These solid tumours usually begin within a few years of a young woman beginning menstruation and under the influence of the ovarian hormones (estrogen and progesterone) they continue to grow while a woman is producing these hormones. Over 50 per cent of women have fibroids in their uterus but most remain relatively small and cause no symptoms or problems. On reaching the menopause, and the ovaries stopping the production of estrogen, most fibroids shrink in size and frequently disappear. The continuation of estrogen following the menopause may allow these fibroids to continue their growth pattern and produce unwanted symptoms such as pressure on the capacity of the bladder, a heavy dragging ache in the pelvis or even induce a uterine bleed. While these symptoms or side effects are rare, the resultant growth of the fibroid may result in the necessity of stopping the HRT or having the fibroids removed at a hysterectomy.

Conditions such as breast cancer, endometriosis and fibroids may be made worse by the use of an estradiol-based therapy, so caution must be taken whenever a woman with such a diagnosis enquires about the use of HRT. However, there is never a time in a woman's life when she must be precluded from using HRT. It is for a woman herself to choose whether she has HRT or not and every healthcare adviser has a responsibility to discuss the benefits and potential adverse findings associated with estrogen and progestogen therapy for a woman following either breast cancer, endometriosis or a known fibroid.

A decision can only be made by a woman herself, based on the risk likely to occur, or the increased likelihood of an adverse event following the use of estradiol versus the degree of distress being experienced when estradiol is not used.

Health practitioners do not have the right nor do they have the authority to withhold HRT, but they do have an obligation to explain carefully the potential adverse outcome following the use of HRT following the diagnosis of an estrogen-dependent disease.

No matter what the disease, there are always exceptions to the advice to avoid HRT and the long-term results are not always adverse – the outcome may actually lead to a health benefit, even following breast cancer.

Summary

- A woman who has been treated for breast cancer or who has endometriosis or a fibroid may be advised by her doctor to avoid the use of HRT for symptoms of the menopause. This advice is usually given because of the risk that hormone therapy may have a detrimental effect on the long-term outcome of the disease.
- HRT after breast cancer depends on the type of cancer – the stage of cancer, the grade of the cancer, and the hormone receptor status of the cancer – and the results of the treatment for that cancer.
- There is never a situation where a woman who has had breast cancer should be precluded from being offered a form of hormone therapy.
- Some studies have shown that women who have used HRT after breast cancer have not had an increased risk of recurrence or death.
- A woman with endometriosis can have estrogen to relieve her symptoms of the menopause if the estrogen is accompanied by a progestogen in a dose sufficient to inhibit the growth of endometriotic deposits.

- After the menopause and the subsequent loss of estrogen, fibroids frequently disappear, so the use of estrogen therapy for a woman with fibroids may enable a fibroid to grow.
- Conditions such as breast cancer, endometriosis and fibroids my be made worse by the use of an estradiol-based therapy, so caution must be taken whenever a woman with one of these conditions requires HRT.
- It is for a woman herself, after careful consultation, specialist advice and consideration of the risks, to choose whether she has HRT or not.

Section Four

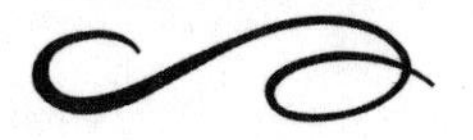

Choices

CHAPTER 15

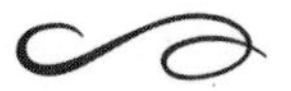

The balance and beauty of ageing

You have to make peace with yourself. The key is to find harmony in what you have.

—Naomi Watts

Ageing is not something that begins just before we discover our first wrinkle or our first grey hair. We begin to age when we are ten or eleven years of age or before we reach puberty. This age is estimated because at this time in our lives, we have less risk of dying than at any other time.

We slough and renew cells in the process of apoptosis. Apoptosis is part of the normal process during growth in which redundant and damaged cells are removed both during embryological development and as we age. Apoptosis regulates the number of body cells, and eliminates many potentially dangerous mutations such as cancer cells. From twelve years of age cells die off not so much because they are not needed but because they have aged beyond usefulness.[120] This is the start of the process of ageing.

Life expectancy is determined as the average of a population's age at death and it is the lifespan of our years from the time of our birth. If there are many deaths of infants and young children in a community, then these premature deaths will lower the average life expectancy of the community, regardless of how long adults in the same community typically live. In Australia, most of the population has a life expectancy rate that has increased by 25 years over the last 100 years. This is due to the fact that the infant mortality rate has fallen because of improved hygiene and medical practice as well as an improvement in our standard of living, sanitation and other community living conditions. As we become aware that there is the possibility of living well into our nineties, or even to become centenarians, we as individuals are obliged through our health and life choices, to be responsible for maintaining our health and deciding how we live in our 'elder' years.

Life is a process where cells continually reproduce, evolve, die and are replaced – four elements found in every one of our stages of growth. We are continually evolving into a new aspect of our self. This is how we grow into the person that we are today. One only needs to look at a child or a flower and look at the stages of its growth in order to see the changes that take place on the journey to beauty and maturity. By the time a woman reaches menopause the changes that have taken place in her have contributed to her wisdom – that of knowing the things that she can change in her life, the things that she can't and the wisdom to know the difference.

From puberty, a girl changes into an adolescent and from then she becomes a woman. She blossoms into a career and motherhood.

In her forties, she begins to experience many changes – her body, her mind and her emotions may begin to behave erratically and it can be a time of huge upheaval. At the time of her menopause, a woman can have an initial feeling of relief but this can often be followed by a descent into mourning for a part of her that is now in her past – the loss of a part of her identity – her perception of 'who she is', 'what her purpose in life is' and 'why' she is the woman she thinks she is. With any loss comes a time of grief and its different stages: the anger, the sadness, the denial, the bargaining, and eventually the acceptance of loss. Then with understanding and wisdom comes new personal growth.

Personal growth is not soft. It can be very hard. However, when the difficulties subside there is relief and a time of reflection out of which comes the search for meaning – why have I suddenly got to where I am now, what is the purpose of my life and how can I create a meaningful and productive life for myself?

Beauty, it is said, is in the eye of the beholder. The subjective or inner experience of 'beauty' can be an interpretation of some part of us that is in balance and harmony with nature and which leads to feelings of attraction and emotional wellbeing. In its most inner and profound sense, we can associate beauty with anything that resonates with personal meaning. So if beauty is in the eye of the beholder – beauty is unique to each one of us.

Nature never allows us to have anything for nothing, and this certainly is true of the menopause. It seems that in order for a woman to move on to a new purpose in her mid-life, she needs to give up her capacity of procreation. Many women say that life in their fifties is fabulous; that they have been able to shrug off the competitive demands of the forties; to begin to laugh at themselves and with others; to think about re-educating themselves; and to revive their sexuality.

Our sexuality is the earthiness of us, what makes us the physical, emotional and spiritual beings that we are. We are sexual beings from the very start of our existence – little babies begin to express their sexuality in their fourth or fifth month after birth and this expression contributes to their vulnerability. Sexuality has the capacity to make and to break relationships, to allow us to feel 'good' about ourselves, and to give us our aliveness. Our sexuality is essential for the survival of the human race. Every generation has a belief that theirs is the only one that enjoys intimacy, but as each generation matures, it discovers that there can be a lot of enjoyment, ecstasy and beauty of sexual intimacy in later life. Self-acceptance is the key to this discovery.

Time does change our body – it no longer matches the images that our sexualised society and its glossy magazines now define as 'perfection'.

The key is to find harmony in what you have.

If middle and elder aged sex is consummated successfully then it can be a far richer and more satisfying experience than in our younger years. If there are difficulties achieving a physical consummation, then a reflection on those difficulties can reveal their source. Is the difficulty a physical one? Is it one of personal relationship? Is it due to fear and anxiety? Is it due to medication? Is it due to the thought that our body image is not 'up to the mark' and therefore 'how' it is, 'how' it acts, reacts and creates love is not up to the mark either? Sensual beauty comes from our heart and from our thoughts. It is the energy that we radiate that is our essence and attraction.

Beauty is in the eye of the beholder.

Like our sexuality, our wellness contributes to our beauty and self-perception. Wellness, as a state of health, is closely associated with our lifestyle. Wellness is not the mere absence of disease. It is a proactive, preventive and positive approach to living – an approach that emphasises the whole person, with an appreciation that everything that we do, think, feel and believe has an impact on our state of health. The secret of our wellness is constant self-care.

To achieve this, our state of health needs to be assessed regularly by a health professional. The regularity of the assessment is determined by our own state of health and is determined by the doctor or health professional who is carrying out the assessment. It is also recommended that a woman have a full gynaecological assessment every year. The routine assessment for a woman of over fifty years generally includes an annual pelvic and breast examination, a regular Pap smear, blood hormone levels, baseline bone density assessment and a mammogram.

Our constant self-care begins with awareness of self. Our body, the food we eat to sustain it, the way we exercise and how we nourish our soul all help to stimulate our awareness. We tend to wait until something is not 'right' with a part of our body before we check it out. We don't consider our head or our toe until we have a headache or a painful toe. We tend to take the health of our body for granted.

We can learn a lot about ourselves beginning with our regular physical medical check-up. Our Body Mass Index (BMI), blood sugar levels, blood pressure, cholesterol levels, Vitamin D status, and our haemoglobin estimates are just some of the results that can jolt us into greater self-care. A general practitioner can do this check-up and make referrals if necessary to other practitioners such as – a nutritionist, a podiatrist, a skin cancer clinic, a psychologist, a sex therapist, a gynaecologist, a cardiologist, a fitness assessor. It is essential for a woman's understanding that the results of any tests are discussed with a general physician so that if necessary, informed choices regarding her therapy can be made.

Dental hygiene and health has a huge impact on the rest of our body. There is an association between cardiac health and the health of our teeth and gums. Bone loss from around teeth results in loss of teeth. This influences how we eat and what we can eat. It influences our nutrition.

As we age, our physical body loses muscle strength and balance. Muscles grow weaker because of the death of some muscle cells and a weakened ability of the remaining muscles to continue to contract. This loss of muscle strength occurs at a rate of 1 per cent with each ageing year.[121] This is why weight-bearing exercise such as walking the 10,000 steps program is encouraged, and for anyone who chooses to attend a gymnasium, there are some that have supervised and safe programs suitable for mature women. Swimming is cardio-pulmonary exercise and participating in aquarobic exercise is not only fun and sociable, it tones and strengthens the body. Local community centres also have exercise programs suitable for mid-life bodies, as well as disciplines such as Yoga or Tai Chi, which not only enhance muscle strength, but also stimulate the brain and encourage the body to maintain its balance. The incidence of falls and fractures is reduced through strengthening muscles and restoring physical balance.

The body's ability to maintain its internal environment in a constant state within physiological limits requires homeostasis of cell function, but balance of the mind and spirit needs maintenance as well. We all have our moments of feeling 'off-balance', and the mind struggles at times to regain its balance. Sometimes we need help with what is concerning us – isolating or hiding our self can perpetuate our discomfort and the only way out of it is to seek help through therapy. Friends can also be a great help because they have often been in the same situation. It is the human condition – it is what we were born for because it is through crisis that we grow and mature in spirit.

You have to make peace with yourself.

Health is a state of complete physical, mental and spiritual wellbeing;

however, a true definition of *good* health is difficult and vague. The word 'health' is derived from the old English *helthe*, meaning whole. We need to try and balance our wholeness – all the essential parts of us that form our identity. We need to know all the parts of our self and to work towards bringing them together in harmony. If we can do this we sustain our emotional welfare, to live happy and fulfilling lives, and to be of benefit for our family and our community. Ageing is the getting of wisdom.

This is the balance and beauty of ageing.

CHAPTER 16

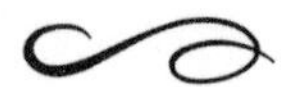

Menopause today

Throughout history there are recorded accounts of the difficulties a woman experienced as she passed through her menopause. In the centuries leading up to the identification of the functions of the ovary and its hormones, particularly estrogen, it was not only the domain of apothecaries, wise women, or witches to determine the mystery of the menopause, it also fell to the realm of philosophers and sages to suggest how a woman should be 'managed'.

The ages of a woman have changed over the last century. A woman now has four ages rather than the traditional three of the maiden, the mother and the crone. Her new age is the mid-life age of maturity – the active, vibrant and creative years which come after her menopause but before she reaches her 'elder' years and which, in the extension of her life span, allows her the opportunity to pursue the hopes and fantasies that she dreamed of during her age of 'mother'.

In our modern time of extended life expectancy, she is a woman of many talents. She looks younger and fitter than her predecessors at the same age; she is much more active than her grandmother was at her age; and she has the potential to re-create herself through further education and the gaining of new skills. She can contribute to the life of our society in ways that even her own mother never had the opportunity to do.

She is also realising her continuing capacity for a rich, beautiful and satisfying intimacy within her marriage or partnership. With the knowledge of modern science and medicine that is allowing her to live a longer life, she can also live this extended life with good health and agility.

The ovary is the only organ in the human body that is programmed to fail. The male equivalent of the ovary, the testis, continues to function for the rest of a man's life, though his sperm count will gradually fall in his later years. This is why a man does not experience the emotional changes associated with the female menopause and the life changes that can come with it.

Menopause is just one day in the life of a woman. It is the day of her last menstrual bleed, and this day is determined retrospectively when twelve months have passed with no further menstruation. It marks the time when her ovary has no more viable eggs. It also marks the time when a woman in transition begins her post-menopausal years.

The post-menopause lasts for the rest of her life. In the law of averages, the rest of her life can last for another 50 years. To adjust to this new reality, a woman might ask herself 'How do I want my life to be in these years?'.

Peri-menopause is the time in a woman's life that can extend from within ten years before the day of her menopause until one year after it. Signs and symptoms of the peri-menopause can begin as early as 35 years of age although the majority of women become aware of symptoms in their mid to late forties. This stage of a woman's life, known as the 'transition' can be a traumatic and confusing period, not only for her, but also for her family, her friends and her work colleagues. This is the time when her failing ovaries are not only running out of eggs, but are also reducing production of her necessary feminine hormones – the ones that help her to remain on an 'even keel'. For many women, it is a time of embarrassing physiological manifestations such as hot flushes, night sweats, disturbed sleep and visible signs of her ageing associated with her lowered levels of estrogen.

The ovaries of a young woman of 20 years produce high levels of estrogen, progesterone and testosterone. Irregular bleeding is usually caused by absent or irregular production of progesterone and this is one of the first signs of the peri-menopause. By the time she is about fifty, not only is her level of estrogen and progesterone almost depleted, but her other ovarian hormone, testosterone, is lessening as well.

It is the depleted level of estrogen in her body that causes a woman the most distress and influences her long-term health. For many women, the fall in ovarian hormone levels does not cause symptoms, but for others the low or depleted or fluctuating levels can lead them into episodes of despair. The time when a woman is most affected by this is during the years of her peri-menopause. These years can be a tumultuous time for her. It is also a time that is not clearly understood by her health-care provider, and often when a woman is struggling with one or more of the symptoms of her peri-menopause these problems can be misdiagnosed by her doctor. The years after her peri-menopause when lack of estrogen begins to affect her bones, her cardiovascular system, and her brain are the 'silent' years of post-menopause. In some instances the distressing symptoms of the peri-menopause may persist for the rest of her life.

Progesterone is a hormone that not only protects the endometrium of a woman's uterus but also influences her brain function by moderating brain cell function, and inducing a calming, sedating effect. In female animals, progesterone is known to induce the 'nesting' instinct, and in humans, progesterone produced in huge amounts in pregnancy induces the psychological and physical changes typical of impending motherhood.

Testosterone, usually regarded as predominantly a male hormone, is also a female sex hormone. Testosterone activates the cells in a woman's brain responsible for her energy levels and her sex drive. Testosterone helps to maintain muscle strength and bone mass, helps relieve menopausal symptoms and depression and facilitates her brain function.

The menopause is merely a point in time. There is one cause of the menopause – the loss of estrogen caused by the depletion of eggs in the ovary. If the lost estrogen is replaced in a woman's body then the effects of the menopause can be reduced. The use of estrogen results in remission of the symptoms and effects of the menopause. It also reduces the risks of osteoporosis, heart attacks, and dementia for a woman in her post-menopause life.

The effects of the menopause are numerous and they can be grouped into two categories.

The first category is the result of the declining number of eggs in the ovaries and the consequent and gradual loss of estrogen that takes place in the years of a woman's peri-menopause. The effects of declining levels of estrogen include the typical hot flushes, night sweats, migraines, sleeping difficulties, depression, mood swings, loss of libido and signs of ageing. A large number of these distressing symptoms have been identified – and they are the ones that inspire a woman to seek help to cope with them.

The second category of effects that follow estrogen deficiency are life-threatening diseases – those of osteoporosis, cardiovascular disease, and Alzheimer's dementia. These problems are usually silent in onset but may present suddenly. When estrogen is no longer available for a woman, then her health can be seriously compromised.

The concern of many that estrogen might be an initiator of breast cancer is no longer as dominant a consideration as it was immediately following the release of the WHI report of 2002. Research suggests that estrogen is a promoter of breast cancer but it is not an initiator of it.

However, the mistaken assumption that hormones cause breast cancer still continues to influence and limit the choices of women and their physicians in how the years following a woman's menopause can be managed. The information contained within this book to dispel this confusion is based on scientific information now available.

Following the release of the WHI report, many women discontinued their use of hormone replacement therapy and switched to the use of alternative and 'natural' therapies. For many, the symptoms of the menopause returned, and for others the resulting long-term effects of this decision are beginning to manifest in problems of their cardiovascular, brain and bone health. For example, over the last seven years, there has been a 50 per cent increase in osteoporotic fractures among women who stopped HRT following publication of the WHI paper. It is anticipated that research will show that a similar increase in heart attacks and dementia will have occurred among women who ceased their HRT.

The results and conclusions from many medical research studies can appear conflicting. The reason for this is that not all studies are equal. It is important to understand the type, the statistics, the quality and the numbers involved in the research performed to appreciate the strength of the results. There are three levels of medical research studies with Level 1 studies being the strongest in design and which attempt to eliminate factors that might give false results.

Level I studies are prospective, placebo-controlled, double-blind studies and are regarded as the highest standard of evidence.

Level 2 studies are observational, retrospective studies comparing two groups or two interventions that have the potential for many biases and therefore require confirmation in Level 1 studies.

Level 3 studies are the weakest of the studies and usually rely on anecdotal reports or small, poorly designed research.

Studies that have been designed to assess regular hormone therapies have generally been Level 1 studies – designed to apply the highest standards to the outcomes. Unfortunately other treatments such as those using 'natural' hormones or alternative therapies have rarely been assessed through Level 1 studies. It is therefore very difficult to assess the efficacy and value of these therapies with any degree of confidence. This is particularly true in evaluating the qualities of these therapies and their effects on diseases of the post-menopause – osteoporosis, cardiovascular disease, and Alzheimer's dementia.

The role of estrogen in reducing the risks of the debilitating diseases of osteoporosis, cardiovascular disease such as heart attack and stroke, and Alzheimer's disease is well documented. It is believed that hormone therapy regimens (HRT) help to reduce the risk of these diseases in a woman's post-menopause years if the therapy is commenced within the 'window of opportunity' – the five to six years following her menopause. There is, at this stage in time, no consensus on how long this therapy should continue. However many women are choosing to remain on

HRT for the remainder of their life not only because of these benefits, but because they feel positive about how HRT affects their general sense of health and wellbeing.

Progesterone is prescribed for a woman who still has her uterus. She must have progesterone or a progestogen with the estrogen in order to protect her endometrium. A woman who has had a hysterectomy can have unopposed estrogen – estrogen on its own.

Testosterone can benefit a woman by improving her muscular strength and bone density but its main advantage is in improving her libido, her drive and her energy levels.

The use of HRT needs to be tailored to the individual. It is not a one-size-fits-all therapy. Often the regimen is just right for her from the beginning of her therapy but it may take up to six months to determine the right products to use. It requires the care of a knowledgeable and sympathetic doctor who has expertise in the management of the menopause to determine the hormone combinations and their dosages.

We live in a world of continuing research and development and our body of knowledge continues to grow and to improve the lives of most of mankind. In spite of adverse statements and publicity regarding HRT, it is now apparent that estrogen therapy, for a young post-menopausal woman, when begun as she passes the menopause (45–55 years) and continued over many years, confers far greater benefits than adverse incidents. Evidence suggests that estrogen:

1. When begun as a woman passes the menopause reduces the incidence of flushes, sweats and insomnia.
2. Improves memory and reduces mood swings and depression in a woman in her peri-menopause.
3. Improves her sexual enjoyment by maintaining the moisture and elasticity of her vagina.
4. Reduces the risk of osteoporitic fractures by 50–70 per cent.
5. Reduces the risk of Alzheimer's dementia by 30 per cent.
6. When initiated during the menopause, has been associated with a reduction in heart attacks and hypertension.[122]
7. When commenced at the time of the menopause and continued for 20 or more years, results in fewer diseases and a longer life than if hormone therapy is never used. Studies reporting on the long-term use of estrogen therapy confirm a 15 per cent reduction in death from all causes. She has an increase in longevity and an improvement in quality of life.[123]
8. Reduces the incidence of bowel cancer and other diseases when administered over a number of years.

For a woman who is unable or does not wish to use HRT because of her perceived risk of breast cancer, but who still wants to reduce the risk of osteoporosis, Specific Estrogen Receptor Modulators (SERMs) offer her an alternative. SERMs are synthesised compounds, that act on specific proteins in target cells in the body and the SERM to be used is prescribed for her individual need. These newer specific therapy regimens offer a woman a reduced risk of breast cancer and osteoporosis.

Menopause symptoms may also be the result of imbalances in the nervous and endocrine system – imbalances in hormones as well as brain chemicals called neurotransmitters that relay signals between nerve cells throughout the body. Neurotransmitters are necessary for proper brain and body functions such as interacting with the endocrine system to enable hormone release and also within the brain and nervous system to allow nerve cells to communicate with each other. When used appropriately, they may help by alleviating the symptoms of the menopause. They do not protect a woman from the increased risks of diseases of the post-menopause – osteoporosis, cardiovascular disease or dementia.

There is a lot of misunderstanding regarding the terms 'natural', 'bio-identical' and 'synthetic' when applied to hormones. 'Bio-identical' refers to the shape of the hormone molecule itself, and a bio-identical hormone has a molecular structure identical to the hormone produced in human females. 'Natural' refers to the source of a product. At present some substances are being marketed as 'natural' or 'derived from plants' yet are not 'bio-identical' to the hormone that is produced *naturally* in the woman's body, nor will these products perform like a bio-identical hormone. 'Natural' refers to something that exists in or is formed by nature. For a hormone to be 'natural' for a woman's body, it must be produced in the woman's body. This is in contrast to a 'synthetic' hormone that is 'synthesised' or produced in a laboratory.

All hormone products commercially available today, including the over-the-counter treatments, are synthesised or produced in a laboratory or pharmacy.

Bio-identical hormones, even though most are derived from chemical products originating in plants, still need to be commercially processed to become bio-identical to human hormones. They are promoted by their proponents as being 'natural' because they are synthesised from plants, and therefore are supposed to be superior to standard hormone therapies. However, the term 'bio-identical' means that the hormones in the product are chemically identical to those produced in the body, but they may not be 'natural'.

Anything that is chemically synthesised is made by combining parts or elements to make a whole. In this sense, the hormones and other treatments described, whether bio-identical or 'chemically altered', are 'synthetic' because they are synthesised in a laboratory as opposed to being extracted from human tissue. Often bio-identical, chemical or other natural preparations are synthesised in the same laboratories as standard hormones used in regular commercial HRT regimens. Of significance is the fact that the only ones that have been rigorously researched and subjected to Level 1 studies are those that are standard hormone replacement therapy.

Complementary and alternative therapies for the menopause do not require a doctor's consultation or prescription, but they are not without risk for the consumer. Some may have no effect at all, while others may convey some element of risk to the user. By relying on these products, a woman is denied full pathology testing, her annual gynaecological examination and screening tests such as mammogram or bone density studies to assess her physiological requirements.

A woman's menopause is part of her ageing process. It is a 'natural' life progression. In our modern age, with technological and scientific advances, a woman is experiencing an extended life and she will possibly live 30–40 years past her menopause but without the advantages of her own estrogen to help reduce her risk of osteoporosis, cardiovascular disease and Alzheimer's dementia. Fortunately, science is refining ways of providing her with hormone therapy so that she can live her extended life with good health and wellbeing.

There is a balance to beauty and ageing. A woman in her years of maturity can re-create herself with education, retraining and a new career. She has the opportunity to develop positive ways of looking after her own health and wellbeing. She can also realise her continuing capacity for a rich, beautiful and satisfying intimacy within her marriage or partnership. With the knowledge of modern science and medicine that is allowing her to live a longer life, she can be … a woman for all seasons.

Epilogue

The year 2011 saw the honour of the Nobel Peace Prize bestowed jointly upon three courageous women – Ellen Johnson Sirleaf and Leymah Gbowee of Liberia, and Tawakkul Karman of Yemen. Their prize motivation was for their non-violent struggle for the safety of women and for women's rights to full participation in peace-building work. You might wonder how this can translate into a book such as this. Well, it is time for women to learn more about themselves, their rights, their freedoms, their possibilities, and how they can enrich themselves for a long and productive life.

Here, the words of Ellen Johnson Sirleaf in her Nobel Peace Lecture,

> *A Voice for Freedom:*
>
> *'If I might thus speak to girls and women everywhere,*
> *I would issue them this simple invitation:*
> *My sisters, my daughters, my friends, find your voices'.*

It is now time for all women to debate how they would like their middle life and elder years to be, and the kind of freedoms that they would like to have.

We encourage you to find your voices and to start talking about the menopause, *your* menopause.

DR BARRY G. WREN
MARGARET STEPHENSON MEERE

Section Five

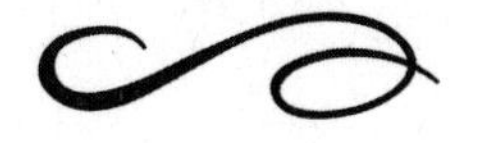

Glossary

Adverse event—is an unwanted and sometimes harmful outcome. It may or may not be related to a medicine, and it is not the same as a side effect.

Amyloid (beta-amyloid β-amyloid) a toxic protein, which eventually destroys neurons. It is derived from an innocuous precursor protein called Amyloid Precursor Protein. The enzyme that converts the APP into the toxic protein is called secretase.

Anti-Mullerian Hormone (AMH)—a hormone produced in the ovary. Johannes Peter Müller was a German anatomist and physiologist who in the 1830s described in detail the development of the Fallopian tubes. In females they grow together in the midline of the pelvis to form the uterus and the tubes. In male embryos, the tubes are prevented from growing into a uterus by a hormone called Anti-Müllerian Hormone, produced in the testes of these very small embryos. This same hormone is produced in cells surrounding eggs in the ovaries of adult women. If there are no eggs present in the ovary, there will be no AMH being produced. This information is very helpful when determining if a woman has any eggs remaining in her ovary, particularly those who have delayed their first pregnancy until late in their reproductive life.

Atypia is a pathological term applied to a cell that has begun to alter its appearance and behaviour as a result of a series of genetic mutations in a chromosome.

Australian Register of Therapeutic Goods (ARTG)—a register of medicines that include a unique **AUST L** or **AUST R** number on the label. This labelling is required for the lawful supply of a therapeutic good in Australia. Where the medicine label does not include an AUST L or AUST R number, then the TGA has not evaluated the quality, therefore the safety or efficacy of the product is unknown. See Appendix 1.

Body Mass Index (BMI)—A measure of an adult's body fat, based on the height and weight (mass in kilograms divided by height in metres^2). A healthy body mass index is between 20 and 25, overweight adults have a BMI 26–30 while obese adults have a BMI of 31 plus.

Bolus—The total amount of medicine administered in a single dose.

Cancer in-situ—A cell that has developed the characteristics of a cancer but is unable to invade or to spread because cell-to-cell adhesive properties and other protective functions have not been disrupted by genetic mutations.

Case-control studies compare a group of subjects (who have a disease), with a similar group of individuals (without the disease) to determine if there are any characteristics that might account for the disease.

Chromosomes consist of enormously long thread-like chains or strands of DNA (deoxyribonucleic acid) incorporating the genes that carry every piece of information necessary for our cells and our body to develop and function as it does. The nucleus of each cell of our body contains 46-paired chromosomes, half of which are inherited from the mother and half from the father.

Cluster cancers—Cancers that occur in a significant number of people who come into contact in closely associated communities such as a workplace or geographical area. They are usually caused by a chemical or a virus, common to all those who develop the cancer.

Cohort—An epidemiological term to describe a group (animal, plant, human) that is being analysed.

Cohort Studies observe a large group of individuals over long periods of time in an attempt to determine if any lifestyle or environmental factors are consistently present to account for the disease or differences in outcome.

DEXA or Dual Energy X-ray Absorptiometry. It is a radiological system to measure the density of bone—it reflects the density of a mineral (calcium) in the bone.

Double-blind placebo-controlled trials is a scientific experiment in which both the subject and the experimenter do not know who receives the therapy being investigated. These trials are designed to avoid bias on the part of the subject or the observer.

Embolus—A term used to describe a mass of material in the blood stream. It usually refers to a blood clot that breaks free and is carried to another part of the body.

Endometrium—the special endothelial cells that line the uterus.

Endothelium—the surface cells lining the inner wall of an organ such as gut, blood vessels, uterus, mouth.

Estradiol (oestradiol)—The primary female hormone produced by the active granulosa cells of a developing follicle in the ovary. It is excreted into the circulation where enzymes degrade it to form estrone. Estrone is further degraded to estriol. Estradiol stimulates growth of the endometrial, uterine, vaginal and breast cells as well as maintaining bone, blood vessel, brain, skin and muscle cell activity. Estradiol is the most important female hormone in much the same way that testosterone is the most important male hormone.

Estrone—a degraded product of estradiol. Its potency is approximately 10 per cent that of estradiol.

Estriol—a degraded product of estrone. It has a potency that may be as low as 1 per cent of estradiol.

Excipient—is an inactive substance used as a carrier for an active ingredient—usually a cream or tablet containing a specific product.

Genes—The protein units of inheritance that dictate every hereditary characteristic of a living organism.

Halo effect—Whenever a new therapy is prescribed for a person, there is often an instant belief, and relief, that a 'cure' has been provided. This belief is a very powerful agent in curing a number of symptoms and the positive influence is similar to the effect of a placebo. Unfortunately, for pathological diseases involving cell mutations, or alteration in the ability of a cell to maintain homeostasis, the 'cure' is not permanent.

Homeostasis (physiological equilibrium) is the term used to describe the balanced activity, normal growth pattern and orderly reproductive potential in living organisms.

Hypothalamus is the neurological centre in the base of the midbrain that is responsible for controlling all autonomous functions of the body by responding to a stimulus by activating a self-preserving hormone response system.

Immunoglobulins are proteins with multiple protective functions. One group on the surface of cells causes cells to stick to each other – maintain cells within their designated site, for example, a breast duct cancer cell remains in its designated site unless there is a mutation in the immunoglobulin, which binds the cell to its normal neighbouring cell.

Menopause is the day a woman has her last menstrual bleed.

Metabolism is the chemical changes in a cell in which various products are broken down to provide new compounds or release energy.

Mitosis is the process of cell division.

Mutation is the term used to describe damage to, or alteration of, a gene during cell division. Over 3 million items of genetic information are divided evenly and pass to the two daughter cells during each cell division, so it is common that an alteration or mistake in a chromosome occurs during the cell replication process. These mistakes or translocations are the mutations that commonly occur and some may produce cancer.

Observational epidemiological studies are relatively quick and cheap research techniques favoured by statisticians who wish to determine if any association exists between an event and an outcome. The two such statistical systems favoured by epidemiologists are the case-control and the cohort studies.

Observational studies are studies comparing groups of subjects who have not been specifically allocated to receive the therapy being studied. Inferences are drawn about possible effects of treatment.

Oestradiol (estradiol)—In the 17th century English physicians 'borrowed' words from French and Italian authors, but thought a number were of Greek origin so spelled them incorrectly. This misuse of the spelling of a number of words has persisted in modern English medical texts when most are of Latin origin (oestradiol/*estradiol,* foetus/*fetus,* etc.)

Peri-menopause is the period of time leading up to and including the twelve months following the menopause. Commonly associated with irregular menstrual bleeding caused by irregular production of ovarian hormones and lasting from the moment the number of eggs is found to be in decline until all eggs have been exhausted in the ovary. Typically it may last three to five years but can be shorter or longer depending on the rate of attrition of eggs in the ovary.

Pessary is a medicated suppository for the vagina or a device to support a prolapse of the vagina.

Pharmacokinetics is a term used to describe the study of absorption and distribution of an administered drug or substance. It involves determining the rate at which a drug action lasts, when it begins to take effect, and the chemical changes it induces in the cell as well as its rate of metabolism, its excretion and the metabolites being produced.

Phyto-estrogens are plant-derived chemicals with estrogen-like activity.

Placebo is a medical term for a medicine that performs no physiological function but may benefit the patient psychologically. It is taken from the Latin meaning 'I shall be pleasing, acceptable'. It is important to realise that the use of a placebo alone, as a therapeutic agent, results in remission of symptoms such as flushes in over 50 per cent of women but even if there was some remission of flushes, would not have any long-term health benefit. Therefore, any drug, which is used to treat problems in the post-menopausal phase of a woman's life must demonstrate success, by a statistically significant margin, in excess of 50 per cent before it can be considered to be of value.

Progesterone is the steroid hormone produced in the ovary by granulosa cells of a corpus luteum. Progesterone is essential for inducing a secretory action in the endometrium and it is necessary to support implantation of an embryo and sustain a pregnancy. It stops uncontrolled growth of endometrial and breast cells and reduces the risk of developing cancer of the uterus.

Progestin is the word used in the United States to describe a synthesised progestogen.

Progestogen is a synthesised chemical substance that is capable of combining with a progesterone receptor and which exerts an action similar to that produced by natural progesterone.

Prophylaxis is the prevention of an event that is likely to occur if no intervention takes place.

Putative describes a substance that is commonly present and reputed to have some effect or influence, but evidence for an action is not obvious or identified. It is a term used in regard to genetic mutations, which have been identified in cells but which do not have a readily recognised role or purpose.

Putative genes are often referred to as genetic 'junk' but have been recently identified as essential to maintain normal homeostasis in cells.

Randomised controlled studies are clinical research studies involving subjects who are randomly allocated to a treatment group or a control group before the trial begins.

Relative Risk is a statistical term to describe the ratio of the chance of a disease developing among members of a population exposed to a factor, compared with a similar population not exposed to the factor. A relative risk (RR) of 1.0 (one) indicates no difference between two groups whereas an RR greater than 1. 0 (for instance 3.30) indicates a three times increased risk while an RR of less than 1 (for instance 0.78) suggests a lower risk. The reliability of any quoted Relative Risk depends on the number of individuals in the study and statistical validity)

Re-uptake refers to the re-absorption of excess neurotransmitter molecules in a synaptic cleft by a sending neuron.

Risk-factor epidemiology is an observational, statistical study of the causes of diseases such as cancer and heart disease.

Secretase—is the enzyme that converts benign amyloid precursor protein into the toxic β-amyloid.

Serotonin—a neurotransmitter known to regulate ageing, learning and memory.

Side effect—a known unintended effect of a medicine or treatment.

Standard deviation is a statistical term to describe how much variation exists from the average mean value of a particular sum of events. It is used to provide some indication as to the variability of a particular figure or result that is different from the average.

Substrate is any substance, which, by itself has no major identified action but which can be converted by an enzyme to produce an active substance.

TAU are proteins that stabilise microtubules in neurons. They are abundant in the central nervous system and less common elsewhere.

The window of opportunity refers to the five to six years following cessation of menstrual bleeding and before loss of estrogen results in irreversible changes to dependent organs or tissue.

Thrombosis is a fibrinous clot that forms in and obstructs a blood vessel.

Troche—a lozenge containing one or more hormones that can easily enter the circulating blood stream after passing through the mucous membrane of the mouth. The advantage of a troche for hormone therapy is its easy absorption and the fact that the hormone does not need to pass through the liver.

Unopposed estrogen is estrogen used alone, that is, without progesterone.

Acronyms

ABS—Australian Bureau of Statistics
AMH—Anti-Mullerian Hormone
AMS—Australian Menopause Society
APP—Amyloid Protein Precursor
BMD—Bone Mineral Density
CVD—Cardiovascular Disease
DEXA—Dual Energy X-ray Absorptiometry
DHEA—Dehydroepiandrosterone
FAI—Free Androgen Index
HERS—Heart and Estrogen/progestin Replacement Study
HRT—Hormone Replacement Therapy
HSDD—Hypoactive Sexual Desire Disorder
IDSMB—Independent Data and Safety Monitoring Board
IMS—International Menopause Society
IUD—Intra uterine device
MPA—Medroxyprogesterone acetate (Provera)
MWS—The Million Women Study
NAMS—North American Menopause Society
PMT—Pre-Menstrual Tension
SERMs—Specific Estrogen Receptor Modulators
SHBG—Sex Hormone Binding Globulin
TAU—proteins that stabilise microtubules in the neurons of the brain
TGA—Therapeutic Goods Administration
WHI—Women's Health Initiative Study
WHIMS—Women's Health Initiative Memory Study

Appendices

Appendix 1

Therapeutic goods administration (TGA)

Any Australian registered drug or product claiming to have therapeutic value and that has been validated by the TGA, may be identified by 'AUST R' on the product label.

Unregistered therapies must have 'AUST L' on the product label in order to differentiate these products from registered ones.

What does TGA approval of medicines mean?

John McEwen, Principal Medical Adviser, Therapeutic Goods Administration, Canberra

The Therapeutic Goods Administration is a Commonwealth Government agency that regulates medical devices and drugs. Prescription medicines and over-the-counter medicines, which meet Australian standards of quality, safety and efficacy are included on the Australian Register of Therapeutic Goods. Medicines may be registered or listed. Registered products are thoroughly evaluated and are labelled with an AUST R number. Listed products, such as complementary medicines, do not have to undergo the same assessments and are labelled with an AUST L number. They are not routinely evaluated before marketing, but are subject to a random audit after listing. Some medicines, such as those compounded for individual patients, are not regulated.

Key words: drug industry, drug regulation. (Aust Prescr 2004;27:156–8)

Appendix 2

Since the invention of synthetic hormones in the 1930s and the development of the Marker Degradation process allowing the pharmaceutical industry to produce bio-identical hormones, a number of pharmaceutical companies have competed to produce better and safer regimens of therapy to treat a woman in the post-menopause phase of her life. The following catalogue of hormone therapies includes hormone products commonly used in Australia. Most of these products are available internationally but may have different names or slightly variable formulations in different countries, but all contain either bio-identical estradiol or synthesised estrogens alone or combined with either bio-identical progesterone or a synthesised progestogen.

Oral hormone preparations—estrogen/progesterone/progestogens

ANGELIQ 1/2 is a low dose continuous combined hormonal therapy regimen containing 1mg of estradiol plus 2mg of drospirenone to be taken every day. Drospirenone is a relatively new progestogen that has similar properties to natural progesterone and as such it has anti-androgenic (anti-masculinising) activity as well as salt and water excreting properties. Because of these actions it would appear to be an ideal progestogen to use in therapy regimens to treat postmenopausal women who have problems of fluid retention, hypertension or excess hair growth. The amount of estradiol in Angeliq 1/2 is usually sufficient to keep menopausal symptoms under control, to inhibit cardiovascular changes and reduce the risk of osteoporosis while the amount of progestogen is sufficient to inhibit endometrial cell growth and reduce the possibility of breakthrough bleeding. It is one of the new generation hormone therapy regimens introduced to enhance the overall beneficial outcome for post-menopausal women without inducing unwanted side-effects.

ESTROFEM is an oral tablet of estradiol with hemihydrate as a stabiliser molecule to reduce rapid degradation by enzymes in the gut and liver. It is dispensed in 1mg or 2mg packs. Because its action is identical to the human 17-β estradiol it is able to simulate all the functional actions of the natural estrogen produced by the ovary. It is prepared in attractive calendar dial packs of 28 tablets which help remind a woman when to take the next tablet. If used for a woman who still has her uterus, then a progestogen must be added to the therapy regimen.

FEMOSTON is a sequential oral therapy regimen, which contains estradiol 2mg to be used alone for 14 days followed by estradiol 2mg with dydrogesterone 10mg for the next 14 days. It is a regimen recommended for a peri-menopausal woman who suffers from problems of hormone dysfunction and who wishes to continue having regular withdrawal bleeds. It cannot be used as a contraceptive.

KLIOGEST is a continuous combined oral therapy regimen in which each tablet contains 2mg of estradiol and 1mg of norethisterone acetate. Like Estrofem, Kliogest is also dispensed in a calendar dial pack and provides sufficient estradiol to provide relief from menopausal symptoms. Kliogest is ideal to treat women in the immediate post-menopausal phase of life when a slightly higher dose of hormonal therapy is often required to control the disturbing symptoms which manifest themselves during the transition from normal physiological levels of hormones to the time when very little is produced.

When menopause symptoms are well controlled (or if break-through bleeding becomes a nuisance), prescribing Kliovance, which contains half the amount of hormones may be more suitable.

Kliogest has a dose of progestogen (norethisterone 1mg), which is similar to the amount found in a number of oral contraceptives. It can be used during the peri-menopause with the advice that it is also capable of inhibiting ovulation and therefore is equivalent to a contraceptive. In fact, (although not recommended by the manufacturing pharmaceutical company) Kliogest, administered every day to pre-menopausal women, not only inhibits the hypothalamic/pituitary/ovarian cascade of hormones, but by suppressing ovulation, restricts endometrial growth and as a result stops menstruation. This can be a blessing for those women who suffer from menstrual pain or heavy blood loss but who do not wish to have a surgical intervention (such as a hysterectomy) to treat the menstrual symptoms.

KLIOVANCE is a continuous combined oral estradiol and norethisterone acetate regimen, similar to Kliogest, dispensed in a calendar dial pack, but with a dose of both hormones that is half the strength of Kliogest. It contains 1 mg of estradiol and 0.5mg of norethisterone acetate. Because of the lower dose of both estradiol and progestogen, there are fewer adverse problems, but the lower level of estradiol and progestogen may not always control severe flushes and sweats.

TRISEQUENS—As the name implies, this is an oral regimen composed of three different doses of estradiol and norethisterone presented in a calendar dial pack containing 28 tablets. Each pack contains 12 tablets of estradiol at 2mg strength followed by 10 tablets of estradiol 2mg combined with norethisterone acetate 1mg, then 6 tablets of estradiol only at 1mg. This triphasic pattern of hormones is designed to mimic the regular cyclic production of hormones in normal menstruating women. It is a very acceptable regimen of therapy for women experiencing menopausal symptoms during the peri-menopausal years. The only adverse problems related to this regimen are the potential to continue a slight menstrual bleed with associated symptoms and on occasions, to produce mastalgia (painful breasts).

PREMARIN—(conjugated equine estrogen) is a complex of equine estrogens extracted from the urine of pregnant mares and was first introduced in 1941. Because it was the first of the 'natural' estrogens, Premarin became the market leader in the USA for estrogenic hormone therapy regimens. Composed of thirteen or more equine estrogens, at least half of its estrogenic compounds are identical to those produced by a woman. Most of the recent studies in the USA which reported adverse effects of hormone therapy, and which caused alarm in the community, were conducted with Premarin as the estrogen. Premarin is sold in tablets of 0.3mg and 0.625mg. Like all other estrogens, when used for a woman who still has her uterus, a progestogen should be added for at least twelve days each month.

PREMIA 5 CONTINUOUS—This combined regimen comes in a pack containing both Premarin 0.625mg and medroxyprogesterone acetate (Provera) 5mg in the one tablet. It provides excellent control of menopause symptoms and the risk of adverse side effects (breakthrough bleeding, mastalgia, etc) following the first three months is very low. It reduces the risk of osteoporosis and other long-term signs of estrogen deficiency.

PREMIA 2.5 CONTINUOUS has a lower dose of medroxyprogesterone acetate (2.5mg) with Premarin 0.625mg in a format similar to Premia 5 Continuous. There is less breakthrough bleeding but an equally good effect on the control of symptoms and a reduction in the risk of osteoporosis.

PROGYNOVA (estradiol valerate) has a stabiliser compound attached to the estradiol in order to reduce the risk of metabolic degradation by enzymes in the gut and the liver. Like other estrogens, it induces a very positive effect on cells that contain an estrogen receptor (genital tissue, bladder, skin, bone, arteries, heart, brain and the liver). Progynova is presented in packs containing either 1mg or 2mg tablets. If used by women who have an intact uterus, a progestogen must also be used for at least twelve days each month and possibly for every day of the month.

ZUMENON is a 2mg tablet of estradiol, which is suitable for treating women with menopausal symptoms. Sufficient estradiol is available following passage through the liver to have a positive influence on the symptoms of the menopause and therefore it is ideal for women who have had a hysterectomy. However, a progestogen must be added if Zumenon is used for women with an intact uterus.

TIBOLONE (LIVIAL) is an interesting synthetic steroid compound whose molecular structure is very similar to that of the synthetic progestogen, norethisterone. Its molecular profile has been configured so that it has the ability to induce both androgenic and progestogenic activity but once absorbed into the body, enzymes are capable of converting the Livial steroid molecule into estrogen-like compounds.

Tibolone is regarded as a compound with tissue specific activity – it will reduce symptoms like hot flushes and sweats, improve libido and reduce calcium loss from bone but does not stimulate endometrial growth or produce vaginal bleeding. The reason it has such differential activity is due to the various metabolites, which are formed by enzymatic degradation after ingestion.

Within minutes of ingesting a tablet of Livial, enzymes in the gut and liver begin to metabolise the molecule of Livial. Several different metabolites are produced from the Livial molecule, each having different actions on different cells in the human female. Two metabolites (3-OH tibolones) will bind to and activate estrogen receptors in brain cells, bone cells and the vagina. By this means Livial inhibits hot flushes, keeps the vaginal epithelium moist and elastic and protects the bone from osteoporosis. But these same estrogenic metabolites are prevented from activating estrogen receptors in the endometrium of the uterus by another metabolite of Livial, which shows affinity only for the progesterone receptor in the endometrium. By binding to the progesterone receptor in the endometrial cells, the progestogenic effect of the Livial metabolite prevents the endometrium from responding to the estrogenic metabolites. For that reason the estrogenic metabolites of Livial do not induce any growth of the endometrium and therefore there is no bleeding and no increase in the risk of endometrial cancer.

Livial also has an interesting action on sulphatase enzyme activity in the breast. Sulphatase is the enzyme capable of converting biologically inert estrone sulphate into the active estrone. By inhibiting sulphatase activity, and thus reducing the local production of estrogen in the breast, it reduces the stimulus to breast cell mitosis.

Livial is capable of maintaining bone mineral density with a reduced risk of fractures, and, because of its androgenic activity it improves mood at the same time having a positive effect on libido.

The **LIFT STUDY** (2008) involving 4538 women recruited to examine the effect of Livial on bone density demonstrated that, not only did Livial reduce the risk of vertebral bone fracture but women using Livial had 68 per cent fewer breast cancers than those using a placebo. This suggested that Livial was an ideal hormone therapy regimen to control symptoms and provide multiple benefits without increasing the risk of breast cancer.[124]

However, a second study the **LIBERATE STUDY** (2009) in which 3148 women with known breast cancer were given Livial, gave contrary results to those from the LIFT STUDY. Almost 60 per cent of the women had Stage 2, 3 or 4 cancer of which 71 per cent were estrogen receptor positive. Half were given Livial as well as other cancer-inhibiting therapy while the other half took only the routine cancer-preventing drugs. The women who were given Livial for an average of 3.1 years had a 1.4 times increased risk of recurrence of breast cancer compared to women who were not receiving Livial.[125]

The results from this study suggested Livial was a promoter of estrogen-dependent residual cancer and therefore it would be unwise to use Livial for women who had stage 2 (or more advanced disease), with the risk of residual disease being present, and who were known to have an estrogen-receptor positive tumour.

Women were advised that while Livial was excellent in reducing the risk of breast cancer in women without a prior malignancy, it was capable of promoting the growth of cancer in a woman who still had viable cancer cells after their breast cancer had been treated. Livial has been shown to reduce low-density lipoprotein cholesterol levels, to decrease lipoprotein and to decrease triglycerides. While the clinical effect of Livial on heart and blood vessels has not yet been clarified Livial is thought to be beneficial to the cardiovascular system. Livial, therefore, has the unique advantage among hormone therapy regimens of inducing all of the three hormone functions.

Because of these multiple actions Livial is capable of controlling the majority of post-menopausal symptoms without inducing bleeding or endometrial hyperplasia. For women with fibroadenosis in breast tissue Livial is instrumental in reducing both mammographic density and mastalgia (which often accompanies the use of other hormone therapy regimens following the menopause).

Occasionally a woman using Livial continues to experience mild hot flushes after beginning therapy, probably because the inhibitory level of estrogen produced from the Livial is insufficient for her needs. However, apart from such a rare event, Livial will stop flushes, sweats, insomnia and will maintain a moist vagina, while the benefits for a woman using Livial are less mastalgia, less breakthrough bleeding and less risk of breast cancer.

The dose of Livial is one 2.5mg tablet daily.

Appendix 3

Progestogens for use with estrogens

Ever since the 1950s it has been known that the use of unopposed estrogen, used by a women with a uterus, is associated with an increased risk of developing uterine cancer. As oral bio-identical progesterone is metabolised so rapidly that it does not achieve a level sufficient to stop abnormal growth of the endometrium, synthetic progestogens are used instead. By the 1970s the use of a progestogen for 12 or more days each month completely eliminated the increased risk of uterine cancer so that HRT could once again be administered.

For most of the past 50 years synthetic oral progestogens have been used, both by mouth or absorbed through the skin.

Medroxyprogesterone acetate (MPA - Provera)

This compound is derived following manipulation of a steroid molecule containing 21 carbon atoms (a C-21 compound) and is used widely in the USA in doses ranging from 2.5mg daily up to 1500mgm daily. The higher doses are often prescribed to reduce the rate of growth of breast cancer cells, whilst 2.5mg and 5mg doses are used in combination with an estrogen for treatment of the menopause. Provera is available either as a tablet by mouth or as an injection (Depo-Provera). It is a relatively weak progestogen so higher doses may need to be prescribed to inhibit growth of the endometrium. These higher doses may be associated with more adverse symptoms (bloating, weight gain, headache, etcetera) than are found with low-dose but more potent progestogens.

Norethisterone acetate—Primolut-N

This is a steroid compound containing 19 carbon atoms. This progestogen is derived by manipulating the testosterone molecule and is therefore regarded as an androgenic (male-promoting) progestogen. As such it may occasionally cause some androgenic effects such as oily skin, acne and hair growth. Because it is extremely potent at inhibiting endometrial proliferation when given continuously, a low dose only needs to be given to suppress endometrial cell activity.

Norethisterone can be prescribed as a tablet of Primolut-N (5000 micrograms), or as one of the progestogen only oral contraceptives (Noriday, Micronor 350 micrograms). It is the progestogen of choice for a number of HRT regimens (as well as for oral contraceptives) and is found in commercial packs combined with estradiol (Kliogest, Kliovance or Trisequens) or added to a transdermal patch (Estalis, Estracombi). Because its chemical structure is very similar to both tibolone (Livial) and testosterone, it exerts not only a progestogenic action but may have some androgenic influence before being enzymatically degraded to an estrogen-like metabolite. Therefore, not only does norethisterone produce beneficial progestogenic effects on the endometrium, but it has also been shown to suppress hot flushes, improve bone density and induce a moist, elastic vagina when prescribed as a single therapy. Conversely, it may also induce adverse effects by raising blood lipids, increasing blood pressure and inducing an oily skin or an increase in acne. It may also have an adverse effect on metabolism and result in some weight gain.

Levonorgestrel

This is another androgenic progestogen that is an even more active C-19 compound than is norethisterone and for its weight is many times more potent than medroxyprogesterone acetate (Provera) at suppressing the endometrium. Because of the high potency, a very low dose only need be prescribed to achieve suppression of endometrial growth. This reduces the risk of adverse side effects such as bloating or weight gain.

Levonorgestrel is used as the progestogen in the IUD (intra-uterine device) known as MIRENA. This IUD delivers levonorgestrel directly to the endometrium with very little being absorbed into the circulation. Proliferation of the endometrium is inhibited while the risk of adverse side effects is almost eliminated.

Cyproterone Acetate - (Androcur)

This is a progestogen that has strong anti-androgenic properties. It is mainly used to treat women who suffer from androgenisation (hair growth, acne, etcetera) associated with Polycystic Ovary Syndrome (PCO). Because it blocks the action of testosterone on receptors within cells, particularly in the skin but also in other tissue such as brain, it has been associated with a reduction in libido, loss of drive and energy and occasionally depression and headaches. It is prescribed in combination with estrogen as a regimen for women who have evidence of increasing hair growth, acne and clinical evidence of adverse effects of abnormal hormone production associated with Polycystic Ovary syndrome.

Drospirenone

Drospirenone is a progestogen that has been designed to reproduce the action of natural progesterone without inducing some of the adverse events, which are often associated with the earlier progestogens.

Drospirenone has the advantage of aiding the loss of salt and water (thus reducing fluid retention, weight gain and hypertension) as well as inhibiting the androgenic (male type) action of other hormones. It is of great advantage to post-menopausal women who suffer from hypertension, bloating, weight gain and hair growth. It is available in a post-menopausal therapy regimen (Angeliq 1/2) combined with estradiol.

Dienogest

Dienogest is the first of the so-called hybrid progestogens. It possesses the unique characteristics of binding to a progesterone receptor in cells to induce responses identical with progesterone, without inducing some of the anti-gonadotrophic actions in the hypothalamus and pituitary, evident with most other progestogens. For that reason it is particularly good at preventing growth of the endometrium without inhibiting the pituitary gland production of FSH and LH.

It does not interfere with the protective effect of estradiol on blood vessels or on other tissue in the body. Popular in Germany where it is manufactured, the HRT tablet containing dienogest is combined with 2mg of estradiol to provide protection without inducing any of the adverse actions that are sometimes associated with the older progestogens.

Dydrogesterone (Duphaston)

Dydrogesterone is a synthesised progestogen which has an excellent inhibitory effect on the endometrium with very few of the adverse effects associated with other C-19 and C-21 synthetic progestogens. It is sold as a 10mg tablet that may be broken in half. A 5mg dose is sufficient to obtain inhibition of the endometrium.

(Unfortunately the pharmaceutical company manufacturing Dydrogesterone has ceased selling this product in Australia.)

Appendix 4

Transdermal therapy regimens—patches, creams, gels, sprays

Oral hormone therapy or medication by mouth results in 90 per cent of the hormones passing from the stomach and small intestines directly to the liver where estradiol increases the activity of liver cells. This may have some adverse consequences (for example, increasing clotting factors, Sex Hormone Binding Globulin). Also liver enzymes may increase the metabolic breakdown of the estradiol thus reducing the effect of it. Transdermal systems, where hormones are absorbed through the skin and mucous membranes, were developed to avoid the problems of oral therapies. Products available are listed below:

CLIMARA is a matrix patch containing estradiol mixed with the adhesive. The patch is made in three sizes, which delivers estradiol through the skin with an average absorption of either 50, 75 or 100 mcg daily of bio-identical estradiol, from the different size patches. The advantage of the Climara patch is that it needs to be changed only once weekly. The main disadvantage is that some women experience skin reactions to the prolonged (seven-day) application of the patch, and when progestogen is required, it must be taken by mouth as an additional daily therapy table.

ESTALIS CONTINUOUS is a matrix transdermal patch incorporating both estradiol and the synthetic progestogen, norethisterone. There are two different doses of the Estalis Continuous Patch. Estalis Continuous 50/140, releases estradiol into the circulation from a patch providing 50mcg of estradiol with 140mcg of norethisterone daily. This combination is capable of inhibiting most menopause symptoms while the progestogen is sufficient to inhibit any endometrial growth. Generally there is no bleeding with Estalis Continuous 50/140.

Estalis Continuous 50/250 also has estradiol at a level that releases 50mcg of estradiol daily into the circulation, but the dosage of norethisterone is increased to release more progesterone daily in order to be more effective to inhibit growth of the endometrium.

Estalis Continuous matrix patches are designed to be changed twice weekly. The advantage of the combined continuous patch is that it has adequate levels of both estradiol and a progestogen in the one patch, making the use of this hormone regimen convenient and effective. The disadvantage is that the dosage regimen is fixed. If any problems arise, such as breakthrough bleeding, a satisfactory result can be achieved by cutting the patch in half. This reduces both the amount of estrogen and the progestogen being absorbed and thus reduces the action on the endometrium, but it is usually able to maintain control of most symptoms without compromising the beneficial effect on the genital and bladder tissue.

ESTALIS SEQUENTIAL are patches that are made in two different sizes. For two weeks, the matrix patch being applied to the skin contains estradiol only, capable of releasing 50mcg of estradiol only each day. For the third and fourth weeks of the month, the matrix patch provides both estradiol 50mcg and nor-ethisterone 140mcg or 250mcg daily. The sequential matrix patch is changed twice weekly and provides peri-menopausal women with the amount of hormones capable of inducing a regular bleed each month. The drawback is that these regular bleeds occur at the time in a woman's life when she would like to avoid having periods altogether.

ESTRADERM PATCHES—These were the first of the transdermal hormone patches produced commercially for women. The Estraderm patch is designed with a reservoir containing estradiol in an ethanol base. The estradiol diffuses through a membrane and passes easily through the skin. Two different-sized patches are available, capable of releasing 25mcg or 100mcg of estradiol daily into the circulation. The reservoir patch is changed twice weekly. If progestogen is required, it must be taken orally every day. The advantage of the Estraderm patch is that it needs to be changed twice weekly only. However, the disadvantage is that the patch is large, it may induce skin irritation and it may not adhere to oily skin. Its use in tropical climates is limited by its adhesive capacity.

ESTRADERM MX is a matrix patch in three sizes, which delivers either 25 or 50 or 100mcg of estradiol over 24 hours. As with all similar matrix patches, it requires the addition of an oral progestogen when used for women who have their uterus. It is changed twice weekly.

ESTRADOT is a matrix patch, which is much smaller than all the other transdermal systems. It contains the same amount of estradiol as is found in most patch systems but the size is less than half that in most other patches. Because of the smaller contact area there are fewer problems associated with skin irritation or reaction. The Estradot patch may be prescribed in dosages releasing 25, 37.5, 50, 75 and 100mcg daily, and is popular because of its greater adhesive qualities as well as its reduced size.

When used for women who still have their uterus, it is important to add a progestogen to reduce the risk of uterine bleeding and cancer.

EVAMIST is composed of estradiol in a fluid in a container holding about 85 measured doses which can be sprayed directly on to the skin of the body or limbs (not on the breasts). It is used once a day and inhibits flushes and menopausal symptoms in over 80 per cent of women using the spray. The spray is applied to the skin as a measured dose and like all other estrogens is easily and rapidly absorbed without being degraded by enzymes in the gut or the liver.

Unfortunately, although developed in Australia and available in the USA, it is not yet licensed by the TGA for sale in Australia.

SANDRENA GEL is a gel containing 1gm of estradiol that is rubbed on to the skin once each day. Most women find the gel to be slightly sticky following the application, so it is best to apply the gel last thing before going to bed. The gel should be rubbed into the skin over an area about the size of the palm of the hand. Because it contains estradiol only, a progestogen must be taken by mouth by those women who have a uterus. The major advantage of Sandrena Gel is that there are very few problems related to skin irritation or of an oily or sweaty application site and, because it is a transdermal gel, the estradiol absorbed from the gel bypasses the gut and liver, thereby avoiding any adverse effects involving the gut or the liver. The disadvantages are few and of minor consequence. It requires a daily application of the gel and although this produces a sticky area for a few minutes, once the gel has dried no adverse effects occur.

NATRAGEN CREAM contains bio-identical estradiol in a 50g tube. The appropriate dose required to control symptoms can be titrated by carefully measuring the dose necessary to suppress flushes, sweats and other menopausal symptoms. It is available by application with a prescription to the manufacturer (Lawley Pharmaceuticals – West Australia). It can be applied to the skin and provides adequate absorption with inhibition of most menopausal symptoms, but no clinical research studies are available to determine if the levels provide bone and cardiovascular system protection. If the uterus is still present, progestogen must be administered by mouth.

Appendix 5

SERMs

Specific estrogen receptor modulators (SERMS) are synthesised compounds that are capable of turning on or turning off a co-regulator for one of the two estradiol receptors withing the nucleus of the cell. SERMs are designed to modify the complex receptor activity in estrogen-dependent cells. The receptors are either estradiol α-receptor (α-ER) or estradiol β-receptor (β-ER). Estrogen-dependent cells contain both of these receptors with each receptor initiating a different action in the same cell at the same time. Some cells will have predominantly α-estrogen receptors or β-estrogen receptors present and SERMs initiate different responses from within the same cell or from different cells depending on the availability of the different protein receptors and co-regulators. The co-regulator controls the type of response of the estrogen receptor. Co-regulators may stimulate or inhibit the response in the cell.

SERMs may provide a substitute therapy for menopausal women who are at risk of, or who have had, estrogen-dependent cancer.

The following is a list of current SERMs, but new SERMs are being produced regularly in an attempt to develop the perfect target-specific product that will produce the best positive activity without inducing any harmful side-effects.

CLOMIPHENE (*Clomid*) is one of the 'oldest' of the SERMs still in active medical service. Clomiphene is an anti-estrogen, which, by blocking the effect of estrogen on the cells in the hypothalamic region of the brain, causes the hypothalamus to interpret the blockage of estradiol as a state of post-menopausal estrogen deficiency. As a result the hypothalamic neurogenic cells, in an attempt to increase and maintain a reasonable level of estrogen for the needs of the body, increases their stimulus to the pituitary, which in turn increases the discharge of follicular-stimulating hormone (FSH) from the pituitary. The increase in follicular stimulating hormone improves the possibility of the ovary producing a follicle containing a viable egg and this effect is used widely to improve the ability of women to ovulate and achieve a pregnancy. Clomiphene was introduced in the 1960s to treat women with breast cancer but because of an increase in flushes and sweats, has not been employed to treat cancer in post-menopausal women.

TAMOXIFEN was another of the early designer SERMs. Introduced during the 1960s, it is still in wide use 50 years later. Tamoxifen stimulates β-ER in bone to preserve calcium and protect against osteoporosis but it also stimulates growth of cells in the uterus, while exerting an antagonist action on α-ER in the breast.

Its action is thought to be mainly as an inhibitor of estradiol α-receptors (in the breast) while it is capable of activating other cells containing β-estradiol receptor (such as bone, vagina and endometrium).

Evidence is abundant that Tamoxifen will reduce the risk of recurrence of established breast cancer by about 30 per cent and reduce the chance of developing a new breast cancer by up to 50 per cent. The main problems when using Tamoxifen are an increase in the frequency and severity of hot flushes, the promotion of endometrial cell proliferation (because of its stimulating effect on β-receptor) leading to break-through bleeding, with an increase in the risk of uterine cancer. Tamoxifen has been used extensively in the management of women with breast cancer, either to reduce the risk of developing cancer in the women thought to be at risk, or to inhibit the stimulation of estrogen in women who have developed breast cancer. Women who use Tamoxifen have double the risk of endometrial cancer than do women of similar age who do not use this therapy.

RALOXIFENE *(Evista)* has agonistic (stimulating) effects on some estrogen receptors and antagonistic (inhibitory) effects on other estrogen receptors. Raloxifene blocks the process that generates growth of cells in breast and uterus, while at the same time promoting beneficial activity in bone cells. Because of this unique action, Raloxifene reduces the risk of breast cancer, reduces the risk of uterine bleeding and endometrial cancer, but increases the bone calcium content and thus reduces the risk of fracture.

In several large studies conducted over three to five years, Raloxifene was shown to increase the amount of calcium in the spinal column by 1.5–2.5 per cent and reduce the risk of vertebral fractures by 30–50 per cent.

Raloxifene reduces the risk of spinal fracture by up to 50 per cent but does not appear to be as effective in reducing the incidence of hip fracture. While Raloxifene does increase calcium deposition in the neck of the femur the incidence of hip fracture in major clinical studies was not improved by its use.

The major advantage in the use of Raloxifene is that it inhibits α-estradiol receptors in breast or uterine cells so cancer in these two sites is prevented or less likely to develop or grow when it is being administered. Through eight years of a study involving over 7000 postmenopausal women, Raloxifene was associated with a significant reduction in the overall risk of breast cancer (HR = 0.42) and this was particularly evident regarding the development of estrogen receptor-positive cancers (HR = 0.24)[126] It also inhibits the deposition of cholesterol in arteries and therefore may reduce the risk of heart attacks.

A study involving almost 20,000 women who took either Tamoxifen (Nolvadex) or Raloxifene (Evista) was published in 2006. The use of raloxiphene resulted in a similar reduction in the risk of breast cancer as with Tamoxifen but with the added benefit of a reduction in uterine cancer and thrombosis.

Raloxifene is a very popular drug to use in order to reduce the risk of osteoporosis without the increased risk of breast cancer associated with regular hormone therapy.

Raloxifene reduces the risk of vertebral fractures and breast cancer, and possibly reduces cardiovascular events as well as reducing the risk of endometrial cancer. However, it does not reduce hot flushes and other menopausal symptoms such as psychological disturbance, erratic behaviour, emotional outbursts or memory loss. Unfortunately, it has also been associated with an increased risk of thrombosis and stroke in women who have increased cardiovascular damage.

BAZEDOXIFENE is a non-steroidal selective estrogen receptor modulator (SERM), which promotes activity of β-estradiol receptor, and which has been designed for the prevention and treatment of osteoporosis. It has been shown to have a very favourable effect on preventing bone loss and in reducing the risk of fractures as well as improving the lipid profile (lowering LDL cholesterol and raising HDL levels) but with the added advantage of being a potent antagonist (inhibitor) to endometrial proliferation and breast cell activity. While this compound has many advantages it does not inhibit hot flushes, sweats or a dry vagina, so when it is used alone it is not effective in treating the vaso-motor menopausal symptoms, which bother a large number of post-menopausal women.

To obtain the advantage of the beneficial effect of Bazedoxifene on bone formation as well as utilising the inhibitory influence on uterine and breast cells it was decided to add an estrogen to the Bazedoxifene. As a consequence clinical trials have been conducted using Premarin 0.625mg and Bazedoxifene at varying dosages.

Bazedoxifene 20mg plus Premarin 0.625mg has been shown to have a favourable clinical profile in women, with beneficial effects on the menopause symptom complex as well as on the skeletal system, with no adverse stimulation of uterine, endometrial or breast cells.

In one trial involving 3397 women for two years, who used Premarin and Bazedoxefine 40mg daily, there was remission of menopausal symptoms, no evidence of endometrial bleeding and there was biochemical evidence that bone turnover was markedly suppressed suggesting that osteoporosis would be inhibited. There was no increase in the incidence of breast cancer.

This new approach to developing improved therapy treatment has been termed the TISSUE SELECTIVE ESTROGEN COMPLEX (TSEC) and Bazedoxifene prescribed with an estrogen such as Premarin appears to be a very suitable combination of therapies to obtain the benefits of HRT without inducing any adverse effects currently associated with regular regimens.[127]

Appendix 6

Neurotransmitter modulators used for menopause symptoms

Brain chemistry plays an essential part in the smooth running of the endocrine system. Neurotransmitters are natural chemicals that conduct messages between nerve cells and are important for the production of sex hormones. Neurotransmitters or transmitter substances are the molecules that are released into the synaptic cleft (gap between nerve connections) in response to an impulse travelling down a nerve (see Chapter 7). They enable nerve cells to connect with each other via their axons and dendrites. If this brain chemistry is disturbed then the brain cells do not communicate properly with each other. There are two neurotransmitter pathways – the first supports the production of inhibitory neurotransmitters that subdue body processes and the second supports the production of excitory neurotransmitters that stimulate them.

A neurotransmitter modulator therefore regulates or adjusts the activity within the synaptic cleft to act on different receptors to enable fast or slow transmission of nerve impulses. If there is a disorder of the action of, for example the neurotransmitter serotonin, then the use of a neurotransmitter modulator (such as the anti-depressant *Prozac*) can regulate the function of it by selectively inhibiting a re-uptake of the serotonin within the synaptic cleft, thereby allowing signals to pass from one neuron to another more easily. This restores the proper action of the neurotransmitter – in this case, serotonin.

The neurotransmitter modulators that have received the most attention as potentially improving flushes and sweats are:

VENLAFAXINE (Efexor) is an antidepressant, which inhibits the re-uptake of the neurotransmitters serotonin and noradrenaline. Some studies in women with breast cancer have suggested that Efexor reduces hot flushes by 50–60 per cent, (similar to the relief obtained when trials are conducted with a placebo) but there may be side-effects for some women, which make its general use for treatment of menopausal symptoms inappropriate. Over 50 per cent of women given Efexor complain of tiredness, loss of interest, loss of libido, bizarre thoughts and general dissatisfaction with the anti-depressant therapy to treat menopausal symptoms. This form of therapy does not reduce the risk of osteoporosis or cardiovascular disease and unfortunately does diminish mental acuity and memory. While there is substantial evidence that some women will derive a reduction in the intensity of, or even obtain relief from, distressing flushes, the use of Efexor as an inhibitor of flushes should not be promoted as a primary treatment regimen for the menopause. This form of therapy to treat menopausal symptoms should only be used if all other therapy options have been exhausted

DESVENLAFAXINE (DVS), which is a derivative of Venlafaxine, has been compared with a placebo in a trial as an inhibitor of vaso-motor symptoms in postmenopausal women. The results suggest that a 100mg tablet of DVS will reduce the number and intensity of hot flushes and as such it may be an acceptable option for women who suffer from mild to moderate vasomotor symptoms, particularly those who do not wish to use regular HRT. However, women also experience the adverse side-effects associated with Efexor and the therapy is often stopped because these symptoms are regarded as worse than those due to estrogen deficiency. More studies are being conducted on this anti-depressant with a view to initiating this form of therapy for women suffering flushes after treatment for breast cancer. To be regarded as a benefit for women it must consistently reduce the incidence of distressing hot flushes by a statistically significant margin. This has not been achieved by any of the studies reported at this stage. Unfortunately it has no beneficial effect on the vagina or on bone density.

LEXAPRO—Escitalopram is another anti-depressant that inhibits serotonin and noradrenaline re-uptake. It has been subject to clinical trials in the USA, and has been shown to reduce the frequency of hot flushes from an average of almost six daily to about four flushes each day. Several clinical studies have supported the concept that Lexapro inhibits the intensity and the number of flushes over a period of twelve weeks and this is of great assistance to the women who suffer from distressing symptoms but because of some medical problem (such as breast cancer) are precluded from using regular HRT. Whether this reduction in flushes is sufficient to justify its use for routine management of the menopause is difficult to determine but it does confirm the impression that hot flushes are associated with an alteration in activity of neurotransmitters in the hypothalamus of the brain, and that further research may produce a drug which actually completely eliminates the vaso-motor symptoms of the menopause.

GABAPENTIN (Neurontin) has been used to treat epilepsy and several studies have suggested that it may also reduce hot flushes. Unfortunately, most of the studies that suggest an improvement have been anecdotal reports, or case-control studies of a small group of women. No major investigations have been conducted. It is not advisable to use this therapy without careful consideration of all other regimens first.

CLONIDINE (Catapres) is a centrally acting adrenoreceptor agonist (stimulant) that is helpful in reducing blood pressure. Several small studies have suggested that women using Catapres have a reduction in hot flushes, but randomised, prospective studies have failed to demonstrate an advantage over use of a placebo.

VERALAPRIDE is a dopamine antagonist that has been developed for control of epilepsy, and several reports have suggested that it may reduce hot flushes. No major studies have reported on its effectiveness compared to placebo.

Appendix 7

Treatment of osteopaenia and osteoporosis

Osteoporosis, and its associated fractures, is one of the most obvious signs of estrogen deficiency. A post-menopausal woman may develop spontaneous crush fractures in her spine, particularly in the upper (thoracic) bones. The resultant dowager's hump is not only disfiguring, but may be associated with severe back pain. The other frequent sites for a fracture of these fragile bones are in the hip (neck of the femur) and the wrist. The best treatment to prevent a fracture is to maintain estrogen therapy together with Vitamin D, calcium and weight-bearing exercise but when bone has been lost and fractures are imminent or have occurred, other chemical treatment such as bisphosphonates and strontium can be instituted.

BISPHOSPHONATES are a group of synthesised compounds, which have been shown to inhibit osteoclasts (the bone cells which absorb bone). To achieve better bone formation while using a bisphosphonate, it is advisable to increase physical activity and to ensure that calcium and vitamin D levels are maintained.

The bisphosphonates may be administered orally or by injection but there are some important cautions that must be followed when using any bisphosphonate. Bisphosphonates bind firmly to calcium to form an insoluble compound, so when taken orally it is important to avoid having any calcium in the stomach till the bisphosphonate has been absorbed. This means it is best to take the bisphosphonate first thing in the morning on an empty stomach, then allow at least 30–60 minutes till the bisphosphonate has been absorbed before taking any other food or drink.

For those requiring a bisphosphonate but who cannot tolerate oral therapy, some bisphosphonates can be administered by injection once or twice every three months while Zoledronic acid can be given as an injection once every 12 months. Clinical evidence shows that bisphosphonates reduce the risk of fracture in spinal bones, the neck of the femur and other bones.

Bisphosphonates inhibit osteoclastic cell activity and therefore reduce the increased absorption of calcium from bone. Some of the commonly prescribed bisphosphonates include:

ALENDRONATE SODIUM (Fosamax, Adronat, Alendrobell, Alendronate). This is one of the most popular bisphosphonates. Although 10mg can be taken by mouth daily or 40mg twice weekly, the most popular method of treatment is to take a 70mg tablet of Alendronate once weekly.

RISEDRONATE SODIUM (Actonel) is another bisphosphonate that, like Fosamax, can be taken daily (5mg) or once weekly (30mg) on an empty stomach.

A 150mg tablet of Risedronate is also available which may be taken once a month.

DISODIUM ETIDRONATE (Didronel) 200mg daily is usually administered daily for two to four weeks followed by calcium alone for ten weeks.

A number of other bisphosphonates (Sodium clodronate, Ibandronate, Pamidronate, Zoledronic acid, Tiludronate) are available but most are used to treat patients with debilitating diseases such as cancer with bone metastases, or Paget's disease or severe osteoporotic fractures. They are not recommended for prophylactic or precautionary treatment of post-menopausal women who have not had a fracture.

Recent reports suggest that the men and women who use bisphosphonates and who undergo oral surgery have a slightly increased risk of developing a very rare condition called osteonecrosis of the jaw. For the women who have no dental problems there is no reason to avoid using bisphophonates.

DENOSUMAB (Prolia) is an injection administered every six months. It acts differently to other osteoporosis inhibiting therapy by binding to the protein receptor that initiates erosion of bone by the osteoclast. When the receptor in osteoclasts is blocked from initiating its normal activation of the nucleus, the osteoclast cell is prevented from mobilising the necessary mechanism that results in the osteoclast eating into, and eroding bone. Research results and clinical evidence suggest that patients receiving Prolia have an improvement in bone content. It is associated with a number of adverse side-effects including osteonecrosis of the jaw.

STRONTIUM RANELATE (Protos) is a mineral trace element. Strontian is a small town in Scotland where deposits of the mineral were first detected. Since its identification the compound has undergone considerable research proving it to be a very useful compound, which not only increases the density of bone, but also markedly reduces the risk of spinal and hip fracture in the women who have osteopaenia.[128] Strontium ranelate inhibits osteoclastic activity in a similar way to bisphosphonates, but it has the added advantage of stimulating osteoblasts, thus increasing the deposition of calcium in bone.

The strength of bone is derived not only from the trabecular matrix in the inner core of the bone but also from the cortical or outer shell of the bones. This is particularly important for long bones such as in the legs, but also for the spinal bones of the back. Research has now demonstrated that Protos increases bone formation in both cortical and trabecular bone to the extent that bone fracture rate in older women is reduced by as much as 50 per cent.

Strontium ranelate is administered as a 2g sachet which may be taken daily for many years, so its use for older women results in the benefit of reducing the risk of fractures of both the spine and the hip, a situation which is clearly more highly prized than suffering a broken hip or experiencing crush fractures in the vertebrae. Strontium ranelate does not have any effect on other symptoms or tissue involved in hormone deficiency (such as flushes and sweats) after the menopause and has very few side effects although occasionally women complain of gastro-intestinal symptoms such as diarrhoea and a skin rash.

SERMs (Specific Estrogen Receptor Modulators) are a group of designer drugs invented to stimulate or to inhibit the various estradiol protein receptors found in bone, breast and uterine cells. The commonly used and prescribed SERMs are Tamoxifen, Clomiphene Citrate and Raloxifene.

Raloxifene is especially popular because, when administered to a post menopausal woman who has no flushes, insomnia or other problems associated with the menopause, will reduce the risk of breast cancer by up to 70 per cent at the same time reducing the risk of vertebral fractures by 30–50 per cent.

A full description of how a SERM works, and specifically the role and action of Raloxifene, can be found in Appendix 5.

CALCITONIN is a hormone, normally produced by the parathyroid gland, and which is commercially available as an extract from salmon (salmon/calcitonin). It has an influence on the modelling/remodelling processes within bone. It reduces osteoclastic erosion of calcium from bone and when used in conjunction with other active osteoblastic therapy, markedly reduces the risk of osteoporosis. However it is not recommended as a prophylactic or as an option to treat women with osteopaenia alone.

CALCIUM, of course, is the essential mineral constituting the building framework of the bone. As such it is important to maintain sufficient calcium intake on a daily basis. The WHO recommendation for calcium is between 800–1200mg of calcium daily. This dose can be achieved by drinking one or two glasses of milk daily or taking a tablet of calcium in addition to the normal dietary calcium.

VITAMIN D (Cholecalciferol)—It is important for post-menopausal women to maintain adequate calcium and Vitamin D levels. The recommended dose is 12.5–25 mg daily (or about 500–1000 IU). For the majority, spending half an hour daily in the sun was thought to be sufficient to convert the base chemical, 7-dehydrocholesterol, into cholecalciferol, but recent evidence suggests that a large number of Australian women are either deficient in Vitamin D or have less than is ideal. So it is now recommended that Vitamin D and calcium be added regularly to the diet of a post-menopausal woman. The level of vitamin D is readily measured by a simple blood test and a normal range should be between 50–150nmol/L.

Vitamin D (Cholecalciferol) increases absorption of calcium from the gut as well as helping to maintain calcium and phosphorus levels in the circulating blood stream. Vitamin D also enhances the efficiency of the immune system and there are claims that Vitamin D is associated with a reduction in the incidence of bowel and breast cancers by as much as 50 per cent and reduces diseases of the cardiovascular system and heart attacks by up to 25 per cent. A number of pharmaceutical companies have developed tablets containing appropriate amounts of both calcium and Vitamin D in a palatable and acceptable therapy regimen.

Appendix 8

Hormones involved in homeostasis (balance) in humans

The following is a list of the more significant hormones involved in maintaining normal homeostasis in a woman. These are only a small number of the hundreds of hormones involved in maintaining harmonious function of the human body and all are coordinated by the hypothalamus.

The hypothalamus of the brain

The hypothalamus is a small area at the back of the frontal lobes of the brain situated behind the nose and between the eye sockets at the back of the nose. It is the homeostatic or chemical balance control centre of the body and is the major integrating link between the nervous system and the endocrine system. It releases a range of hormones to control the activity of the pituitary gland. It also initiates the brain response system, that controls the way that the body deals with changes within our body involving thirst, hunger, ovulation, weight control and also in responding to our outer environment such as to heat by sweating and cold by shivering.

THE PITUITARY GLAND

The pituitary secretes a variety of hormones as directed by the hypothalamus.

- Thyroid-stimulating hormone
- Growth hormone
- Follicle-stimulating hormone.
- Luteinising hormone
- Prolactin
- Oxytocin
- Adrenocorticotrophic hormone
- Anti-diuretic hormone
- Melanocyte stimulating hormone

THE OVARY

- Estradiol, Estrone, Estriol
- Progesterone
- Testosterone
- Anti-Müllerian Hormone (AMH)—secreted by granulosa cells around ova
- Activin—enhances FSH biosynthesis
- Inhibin—inhibits biosynthesis of FSH
- Bone morphogenic hormone—enhances bone development
- Growth differentiating factor

THE THYROID GLAND

- Thyroxin
- Calcitonin

THE PANCREAS AND WEIGHT CONTROL SYSTEM

- Insulin
- Amylin
- Leptin from fat cells
- Ghrelin from the stomach

THE ADRENAL GLAND

- Adrenalin
- Nor-adrenalin
- Aldosterone
- Cortisol
- Androstenedione

THE THYMUS GLAND produces hormones that are involved in the immune system, particularly promoting the proliferation and maturation of T cells.

THE PINEAL GLAND secretes melatonin. It is also thought to inhibit and control gonadal development in children and to be a mediator of menstrual rhythm.

Appendix 9

Hormones and cancer

Many women are concerned about the possibility of developing cancer if they take HRT, so a 'simple' explanation of the sequence of changes that convert a normal cell to a cancer cell follows.

Normal body cells require a messenger in order to carry out many tasks or initiate specific actions. Nerve messengers mediate most immediate and rapid actions in the body, while steady, regular and constant cell function requires hormones in order to achieve and maintain homeostasis.

Normal hormone receptor activity

A hormone is the messenger that tells a cell to perform a specific task. When an estrogen hormone enters a normal breast cell, it 'docks' with its receptor, fitting exactly into the specific niche or cavity in the complex receptor molecule (like a key in a lock, designed to fit only the estrogen molecule). Once the estrogen molecule has 'docked' with its receptor, the receptor becomes active. The activated receptor then enters the nucleus of a cell where it induces cell division (mitosis).

Altered receptor activity in cancer

One of the many changes causing breast cancer involves a mutation to the gene responsible for creating the receptor protein. A mutation in that particular gene may result in the production of a receptor that can initiate cell division without the necessity of an estrogen molecule 'docking' into the receptor (acquired autonomous reproduction).

To avoid irresponsible overgrowth caused by such a mutated receptor, normal breast cells mobilise proteins that suppress or arrest uncontrolled cell division, or even tell the abnormal cell to self-destruct, a process called apoptosis. To overcome these normal inhibitors of abnormal cell division, more mutations must also occur to the many protective inhibitor actions that control an abnormal cell division. It is believed that up to two hundred mutations occur to a breast cell before it becomes so corrupted that it forms a cancer.

Causes of death in women

Following a campaign aimed at making women aware of the need for regular breast checks and mammography, a BBC survey in the United Kingdom in 1998 found that almost 40 per cent of women thought that breast cancer would be the most likely cause of their death. In fact, while 23 per cent of all women will die of some form of malignancy, only 4.2 per cent will die of breast cancer.

Leading causes of death in females, ranked in 2007 by the ABS[129] are as follows:

Table 6

DISEASE	RANK
Heart attacks	1
Stroke	2
Dementia and Alzheimer's disease	3
Lung cancer	4
Breast cancer	6
Diabetes	8
Bowel cancer	10

In Australia, the three most common cancers that cause death in women are lung cancer (5.1 per cent), breast cancer (4.2 per cent) and bowel cancer (3.6 per cent). The Australian Bureau of Statistics reveals that 28 per cent of women will die of some form of cardiovascular disease, and 8.5 per cent will die of stroke. What is often not discussed is that 7 per cent of women will die of dementia.

Age and family history (inherited genetic mutations) are the most important and common risk factors for any woman concerned about developing breast cancer. Having a mother, aunt or sisters with breast cancer, increases the risk over a lifetime by up to seven times while living longer doubles the risk every decade. Hormone replacement therapy increases the risk by only 0.08 per cent annually.

The impression that breast cancer is so common is directly related to the publicity that breast cancer awareness organisations have generated in their education programs. While it is laudable to promote interest in breast cancer, it has resulted in a misinterpretation of the significance of deaths from breast cancer compared to other causes of death.

As we all are living longer and as the risk of developing cancer doubles every ten years, it is inevitable that the incidence of both breast and other cancers will increase as the number of older people in the population increases. Following release of the WHI results in 2002, fear of breast cancer became the major concern for a woman when faced with the choice of either using, or avoiding the use of, hormone replacement therapy. Because of this fear, it is instructive to review the facts regarding the relationship between estradiol (estrogen) and gynaecological cancer.

Cancer is the name applied to a malignant and invasive growth or tumour. It is a group of atypical (abnormal) cells, which multiply autonomously and apparently in an uncontrolled fashion, ignoring signals and physiological messages that dictate the behaviour and function for normal cells.

In discussing the development of cancer, it is necessary to briefly describe the process of cell division and the mutations (genetic changes) involved in turning a normal cell into a cancer cell. To simplify a very complex cellular activity the following terms are some of the terminology now commonly used in the media and in everyday conversation.

Homeostasis

Homeostasis (physiological equilibrium) is the term used to describe the balanced activity, normal growth pattern and orderly reproductive potential in living organisms. This activity is maintained by the actions of hormones and growth factors, in the presence of appropriate nutrition and body cell stability.

Chromosome

A chromosome consists of enormously long thread-like chains or strands of DNA (deoxyribonucleic acid) incorporating the genes that carry every piece of information necessary for our cells and our body to develop and function as it does. The nucleus of each cell of our body contains 46-paired chromosomes, half of which are inherited from the mother and half from the father.

In the chromosome chains the genes are arranged in a very orderly pattern. To package the long strands of protein material, the paired strands of DNA forming a chromosome, coil tightly around each other in a double helix formation. Twenty-two paired strands of chromosomal material are found in the nucleus of every human cell plus two additional strands of chromosomes which carry the sex differentiation genes (X genetic material from the mother, Y from the father) giving a total of 46 chromosomes (23 pairs) in each cell.

Mutations

A mutation is the term used to describe damage to, or alteration of, a gene.

The cells of the body are continually renewing themselves in order to provide for growth and for replacement of old and damaged cells. A cell multiplies by replicating identical copies of itself so that two daughter cells are formed in a process called mitosis. During mitosis the chromosomes with their genetic material, normally split evenly so that each daughter cell receives identical genetic DNA. However, about once in every million cell divisions an accident occurs and there is either a loss of, or translocation of, some genetic elements or some other damage to the protein DNA 'template' in the gene. It is this damage or alteration to the gene is that is called a mutation.

Mutations may be caused by some toxic activity such as X-rays and irradiation, chemicals (for example, those found in cigarettes, asbestos, naphthylamine, etc) and viruses, etc, which damage the DNA, or they may occur spontaneously as chromosomes are splitting when cells undergo division. Only cells in the process of dividing (mitosis) will undergo a mutation. Although a cell may remain static for months or years, when it does decide to divide and multiply in number, the actual process of mitosis is completed in seconds or minutes. The more often that a cell divides, the more frequently will mutations occur.

Genes

Genes are the protein units of inheritance that dictate every hereditary characteristic of a living organism. When a cell divides normally, the exact, identical genetic material is passed to the two daughter cells and this genetic material directs how those two cells will function. A mutated altered gene produces abnormal action within the cell.

Gene Inhibitors

To prevent abnormal cell activity as a result of a mutation, all cells contain inhibitor genes whose only purpose is to block the action of a mutated or altered gene. Cancer will only occur if an inhibitor gene is also altered or corrupted by a mutation.

If the inhibitor mechanism is damaged by a mutation, a repair mechanism normally swings into action to restore the ability of the inhibitor genes to stop uncontrolled cell division. Restoring and repairing damaged inhibitor genes is carried out by repair genes (such as BRCA1 or BRCA2), which are found in the cells of breast, ovarian, bowel and prostate tissue. However, this remarkable repair system may also be affected by a mutation, which renders the repair mechanism ineffective. Mutated or ineffective BRCA1 or BRCA2 protein repair genes may be inherited (frequently among Ashkenazi Jews) or become corrupted by a mutation during cell division. When a person acquires not only a corrupted inhibitor gene but a defective repair gene, the risk of uncontrolled cell proliferation and cancer is increased many-fold.

Genetic alteration (mutation) results in a different set of plans and directions being transmitted to the daughter cells. In some instances, the chromosomal/genetic alteration may be passed, without obvious effect, through many generations to all subsequent daughter cells during regular cell division (inherited change). Although most genetic alterations are inconsequential and cause no harm, or may even result in an improvement, some of the abnormal genetic patterns may be completely incompatible with normal function and their persistence leads to the development of an abnormal cell.

Fortunately the internal defence system of cells is capable of compelling the majority of cells with grossly abnormal mutations to self-destruct (apoptosis), thus eliminating the threat. But if the defence system within a cell is also damaged by mutations, the corrupted genes are able to persist to produce an abnormal (atypical) cell. Cells which initially have only a few inherited abnormal genetic alterations, may, over time, accumulate other mutations as cells continue to divide, and so change the cell activity and appearance that it develops the characteristics and the behaviour of a cancer. This process usually occupies many cell divisions, sometimes requiring many years to accumulate the genetic changes.

It is important to realise that a very large number of mutations are not harmful to the cell or the life of the organism. In fact, beneficial mutations are essential for the advancement and survival of all forms of life. Genetic alterations often result in diversification and improvement in cell activity and function, thus producing the subtle evolutionary changes that have been taking place in humans as well as other life forms for thousands of years.

The majority of mutations that are incompatible with 'good' cell function are destroyed by the built-in protective mechanism that exists in all cells. It is only when mutations have also corrupted the defence mechanism, and the aberrant or misbehaving cells continue to divide, that abnormal cell changes become dominant, producing diseases such as cancer, arthritis, metabolic dysfunction and so on.

In the past it was believed that just one mutation was all that was required to produce a malignant change, but it is now recognised that dozens, if not hundreds, of mutations are involved.

The following is a summary of current findings associated with the development of cancer:

1. All normal cells function with the aid of a complex but integrated internal signalling mechanism, which involves special protein controls that monitor the function and behaviour of an individual cell.[130] Cancer will only occur when the internal signalling system has become corrupted by mutations to the extent the system fails to respond to normal messages.
2. For a cell to become malignant, a large number of alterations (up to 200 mutations) to DNA have been identified in individual breast cancers with a wide variation in the different roles these mutations influence. Of 950 mutations collected from eleven breast cancers that have been examined for mutations, the same 12–15 alterations to the functional roles within a cell have been identified in each breast cancer. It is presumed the mutations causing these changes to the breast cell are the critical mutations essential to induce malignant corruption of the internal cell control system of breast cells,[131] while the majority of the other mutations, which have been identified in most breast cancers are to be regarded as putative (genetic changes which are present – but not necessary to cause a cancer).

3. It is only when mutations damage or corrupt the integrity of the control system that the cell loses its ability to maintain homeostasis (in much the same way that a community which is organised and functions with rules, laws, police, and punishment for offenders may be corrupted by a dishonest group or individual).
4. When a specific number of critical mutations have accumulated in a cell, the alteration to cell activity leads to major malfunction and abnormal behaviour. The cell is no longer capable of responding to normal external messages, nor to the internal control system.[132] It has become a renegade cell—a cancer.

   To understand the cause of a malignant change within a cell, the growth pattern of cancer, the role of the environment, the ability of a cancer cell to invade surrounding tissue, the nutritional requirements and the procedures necessary to eventually overcome cancer we must determine the exact role of all the genetic material in a normal cell and identify how a malignancy has altered the control mechanism. The major areas of cell function that must be corrupted by genetic alterations (mutations) in order to induce a malignant change are:

   a) Autonomous self-induced cell division. To induce a specific action or response within a cell, a messenger hormone or growth factor must pass through the wall of the cell to attach to a ***specific protein receptor*** in the nucleus of the cell (like a key fitting into its particular lock). This interaction between a messenger and its receptor is very specific and essential for normal cell response and behaviour.[133] A good example is the activation of a protein receptor by a hormone in order to initiate the process of cell mitosis (cell division). The intimate union of estradiol with its protein receptor is essential for a cell to initiate the process of mitosis. If however the protein receptor has undergone a mutation, the mutated receptor may be able to initiate the process of cell division without the need for the estradiol messenger hormone. This is autonomous or self-induced reproduction. A mutation of the receptor that results in autonomous cell division is the first step towards tumour growth.
   b) Normal cells do not allow uncontrolled cell division. This is because inhibitor proteins in all normal cells automatically block an abnormal rate of cell replication even if the receptor is mutated. However, if one of the many inhibitor genes in a cell is also corrupted by a mutation, then the normal inhibitory control of cell division is lost and unrestricted growth of a cluster of abnormal cells results, producing a tumour.
   c) If the DNA responsible for controlling cell function becomes corrupted by mutations to the extent that the cell ignores all the usual homeostatic

controls, the abnormal cell is capable of continual multiplication in an uncontrolled way. To protect the body from such tumour overgrowth and invasion, yet another defence mechanism exists. On recognition of abnormal activity within a cell, neighbouring cells send messages which inform mitochondria (responsible for respiration and energy production) within the abnormal cell to initiate the release of caspases and other proteins which force the offending cell to self-destruct in a process known as apoptosis—therefore eliminating the 'wicked' cell. For cancer to become invasive, this remarkable self-destructive system must also be avoided by yet more mutations to the genes that control the self-destruct system.

d) The protective function of telomeres. Normal cells have 46 chromosomes in each cell. When a cell divides to produce two new cells, the chromosomes are split evenly so that each daughter cell contains identical genetic material to the parent cell. Each chromosome has a protective 'cap'—a telomere—which prevents the ends of chromosome strands from being damaged as the cells divide. However every time a cell divides a small portion of the protective telomere (at the end of each chromosome) is lost. Following a finite number of cell divisions, the telomere is so eroded that the exposed ends of the chromosomes form lethal end-to-end amalgamations which precipitate programmed cell death. This system ensures that normal cells are denied the ability to reproduce forever. For a cancer cell to avoid such cell death, it must maintain the telomeres on the corrupted chromosome. Cancer cells achieve this by producing quantities of an enzyme named telomerase.[134] Telomerase maintains and repairs the telomere and thus allows the corrupted cancer cell to reproduce forever.

e) All cell contents are encapsulated within a membrane, which has attachments to, communicates with, and has affinity with its neighbours. Special proteins such as immunoglobulin, cadherin and integrin on the surface of cells ensure the stability and integrity of all organs and tissue to prevent normal cells from migrating from their allotted place. For cancer in-situ (a cancer cell that remains in its original place) to change from a non-invasive state to tissue invasion and metastasis, these proteins must also be altered by a further series of mutations during which the integrity of cell-to-cell relationships is lost. The abnormal cell may then spread and penetrate (metastasise) other areas of the body by direct spread, through blood circulation or through the lymphatic system.

f) Finally, no cancer can grow unless it has an abundant supply of nutrients and oxygen. To supply the extra blood vessels to provide these nutrients, the cancer cells promote a local increase in the secretion of those messengers (angiogenic—or new blood vessel growth factors), which then stimulate the vascular system to increase the growth of new blood vessels. The increase in angiogenic growth factors results in an overwhelming but disorderly proliferation of arteries, capillaries and veins in the vicinity of the tumor. In the future, efforts to defeat cancer will most likely concentrate on genetic manipulation designed to inhibit angiogenesis (the formation of new blood vessels) and thus strangle and starve the cluster of cancer cells before they invade or spread to other sites in the body.

Malignant cell behaviour is caused by an accumulation of many mutations to the protein coding genes that control the homeostatic system of a breast cell.[135] Each individual breast cancer has been identified as having about 150–200 mutations, but up to 950 different mutations have been identified in various breast cancers. However, of these mutations only about 12–15 are regarded as being critical in converting a normal, functional breast cell into a cancer.

Cancer in-situ

As mutations accumulate, the instructions that dictate how a cell should function after receiving a message are altered and the cell begins to behave badly. Not only does it respond in an abnormal manner to normal messengers (hormones) but also it may change both its shape and its relationship to its neighbouring cells. Some cells develop an identical appearance to cancer cells but are unable to invade or to spread because cell-to-cell adhesive properties and other protective functions have not been disrupted by genetic mutations. These cells are known as cancer in-situ.

It is thought that for the majority of women, the accumulation of all the mutations necessary to develop an invasive cancer may take many years, and that a large number of abnormal cells never progress beyond the development of an atypical cell or cancer in-situ.

Whether mutations develop in cells because of the influence of environmental carcinogens such as a virus, a chemical or a some other toxin, or the primary breast stem cells have acquired gene alteration during embryonic development continues to be debated. However, it is likely that in most cancers, a number of the frequently mentioned causative agents, including spontaneous mutations, inherited defects, viruses, toxins, environmental factors, mammographic X-rays, cigarette smoke, anti-oxidants and other chemicals may be involved.

A substantial number of women (autopsy studies suggest between 10 per cent and 30 per cent) are known to have acquired all the genetic mutations involved in breast cancer while they are young and still pre-menopausal, but at least half of these women will never progress to have invasive cancer. Latent breast cancers or cancer in-situ are often detected by sophisticated diagnostic machines. Consequently diagnosis of these pre-invasive conditions often results in surgical procedures, radiotherapy and even chemotherapy for pre-cancerous lesions. However, many experts are now questioning the wisdom of such aggressive intervention, pointing to results showing that some cancer in-situ never invade and sometimes may even undergo spontaneous remission.[136]

Estrogens do not *cause* breast cell mutations, but estrogens may increase the rate of cell multiplication if the cell contains a receptor for estrogen. When malignant mutations have occurred, the use of estradiol may accelerate the rate that the corrupted cell divides and grows into an invasive tumour.

Appendix 10

Assessing research in medical studies

Research studies are not all equal. They must meet certain criteria in order to be classified at different levels of acceptance.

Level 1 studies

These studies (clinical trials) have the strongest design, and they try to eliminate factors that give false results. These studies are described as double-blind, randomised, placebo-controlled trials. The 'double-blind' means that neither the investigator assessing the results nor the volunteer are aware as to whether the volunteers took the placebo (dummy) therapy or the real therapy being investigated. The random allocation of these therapies helps to improve the chance that the groups being studied were similar. Such trials can usually only study one or two regimens and the results apply only to the type of volunteers being studied. The Women's Health Initiative study of post-menopausal hormone therapies was a Level 1 study of women initiating oral combined estrogen and progestogen therapy, mostly many years after the menopause.

Level 2 studies

These studies are called observational studies and are not randomised, double-blind or placebo controlled. Users and non-users of therapies are compared to each other but there is the potential for many biases. Therefore associations seen in observational studies require confirmation by Level 1 studies.

Level 3 studies

These studies are the weakest of all research studies and are usually simple reports of treated cases, without control groups or accurate understanding of the influences that might have affected the results.[137]

Advances in medical knowledge and new approaches to treatment regimens involve contributions from three major research disciplines before a particular hypothesis or idea can be accepted as the correct medical course of action.

When results from all of the three research disciplines are in accord, one can be certain that the conclusion being presented is correct. When there is disagreement and discord between the disciplines then one of the assumptions is likely to be wrong.

The three research disciplines involved in gathering data and formulating new therapy conclusions and advice are:

1. Epidemiology

This is the statistical process during which large amounts of data is collected and reviewed in order to determine if there is an association between an event and a disease. Reviewing such large amounts of information has led to identification of previously unknown causes of disease but has also led to many presumptive hypotheses which have not been confirmed by subsequent scientific study. Unfortunately association is not proof of cause and effect!

Typical examples of epidemiological studies are the WHI in 2002 and the Million Women Study where association has implied that the cause of breast cancer is estradiol.[138] Both of these studies demonstrated an increase in the diagnosis of breast cancer following hormone therapy – the consequences of these reports has resulted in estradiol being blamed as a carcinogen whereas other studies such as the second WHI study in 2004 have suggested that estradiol may actually reduce the incidence of breast cancer.[139]

2. Biological research

This discipline is the study of cell behaviour that often involves exposure to a particular substance or therapy. This form of research is much more detailed, as efforts are made to identify the complex processes involved in cell responses and behaviour. It may involve the study of individual cells in animal models or human tissue and is regarded as the gold standard of research. It is the basis on which clinical treatment is ultimately based. Outstanding and typical biological research studies are:

a) The investigation of the pathological changes found in the breast tissue of women who died of a non-malignant cause. It was demonstrated that over one-third of pre-menopausal women had pathological evidence of cell changes typical of pre-invasive breast cancer.[140] (See Chapter 4)

b) The study involving macaque monkeys to establish the basis for the protective benefit of estrogen on the cardiovascular system.[141]

c) The identification of multiple genetic coding sequences which are present in various forms of human breast cancer.[142]

3. Clinical research

Following suggestion of an epidemiological association and biological evidence regarding a particular hypothesis, it is usual to perform clinical studies over a fixed period of time in order to evaluate the benefits and adverse effects of such an intervention on a group of subjects. An excellent example of clinical research is:

a) The HERS Study demonstrating that when **oral** estrogen was given to older, overweight women with a history of prior cardiovascular disease, it increased the risk of thrombosis and heart attacks.[143] (See Chapter 1)

b) The study proving that estradiol begun at the time of the menopause reduced the risk of osteoporotic fractures.

Endnotes

INTRODUCTION

1 Rossouw JE, Anderson GL, Prentice RL, et al. *Risks and benefits of estrogen plus progestin in healthy postmenopausal women: principal results from the Women's Health Initiative randomized controlled trial* JAMA 2002; 288:321-333

The first major study into the health of post-menopausal women was conceived in the United States of America under the auspices of the National Institute of Health (NIH) and involved recruiting 164,000 women aged between 50 and 79 years to enter a prospective study to be conducted over eight or more years. This ambitious study anticipated gaining an insight into those factors that influenced the health of women after the age of 50 years.

To determine what effect hormone therapy played in the health of these women, 27,349 were allocated to receive either a hormone therapy or a placebo and it is the outcome of the results from these women which has formed the basis of the many reports from the Writing Group who were responsible for reporting the results of hormone therapy in the Women's Health Initiative (WHI) Study.

In the decade since the first paper was published in July 2002, a large number of very significant articles have appeared and conclusions have been drawn based on the outcome of hormone treatment for these women. The first of these articles to appear was written by the writing group led by Dr Jacques Rossouw, but other very significant papers on various aspects of the data obtained from this huge collection of material have been reported regularly (A detailed review of the reported results of the effect of HRT on women aged 50–79 years in the Women's Health Initiative Study in 2002 is available in Chapter 3).

Among the many articles of significance regarding the effect of hormones on health, based on the material gathered from the WHI Study material, published since 2002 are:

Rossouw JE, Anderson GL, Prentice RL, et al, 'Risks and benefits of estrogen progestin in healthy postmenopausal women: principal results from the Women's Health Initiative randomized controlled trial', *JAMA* 2002; 288:321–333

This article was the 'blockbuster' which resulted in a universal condemnation of HRT as inducing a 26 per cent increase in breast cancer, as well as an increase in heart attacks and stroke, with the subsequent advice that women should cease using HRT.

The second important paper from the Writing Group for the Women's Health Initiative Investigators: Anderson GL et al 'Effects of conjugated equine estrogen in postmenopausal women with hysterectomy', *JAMA* 2004; 291:1701–1712 reported that estrogen given alone to post-menopausal women resulted in a 23 per cent reduction in the risk of developing breast cancer—now there was confusion! Which result was true? Or was estrogen no longer the culprit as a cause? Could it be due to the progestogen?

Over the next ten years a number of articles were published from the WHI Writing Group that has produced confusing results and some are listed as follows:

Rossouw JE, Prentice RL, Manson JE, et al, 'Hormone therapy may be safer in younger women? A best evidence review', *JAMA* 2007; 297:1465–1477. With this article the confusion over the 'harm' associated with HRT became more bewildering. The very same group who had advised against using HRT were now stating that if used for younger post-menopausal women estrogen did not induce an increase in heart attacks and may actually be beneficial.

Manson JE, Allison MA, Rossouw JE, et al 'Estrogen therapy and coronary artery calcification' *N Engl J Med 2007; 356:2591-2602.* Instead of using myocardial infarcts (heart attacks) or death as an outcome of hormone therapy use, these WHI researchers measured the amount of calcium deposited in atherosclerotic plaques in the carotid arteries of women to evaluate if estrogen protected against possible damage to arteries.

It was clear that if estrogen was begun soon after the menopause, it reduced the risk of atherosclerosis and therefore had the potential to reduce the risk of stroke or heart attacks in the years to come.

Shumaker SA, Legault C, Rapp SR, et al. Estrogen plus progestin and the incidence of dementia and mild cognitive impairment in postmenopausal women *JAMA 2003;289:2651–2662* and a second article by the same authors: Rapp SR, Espeland MA, Shumaker SA, et al. 'Effect of estrogen plus progestin on global cognitive function in postmenopausal women' *JAMA 2003;289:2663–2672* presented evidence for a relationship between HRT and dementia. It had been reported in previous papers that women using HRT from the age of their menopause appeared to have less dementia and better memory than women who did not take HRT. Because dementia commonly occurs after the age of 65 years, it was decided by the WHI researchers to include only women who were older than 65 years in a study to determine if HRT could reverse or prevent mental deterioration. This was clearly a mistake in selection of subjects, as prevention of a problem should begin long before there is clinical evidence of symptoms.

SECTION ONE: HISTORY, PERI-MENOPAUSE, MENOPAUSE AND HRT

CHAPTER 1 A history of the menopause and HRT

2 Amundsen DW, Diers CJ, 'The age of menopause in classical Greece and Rome', *Human Biology* 1970; 42; 79–8

Bremmer J. in *Sexual Asymmetry: Studies in Ancient Society: The old women of ancient Greece*, (Editors) J Block, P Mason; Amsterdam: JC Gieben pp191–215

Gentile KM, 'Menopause in the Ancient Greek World', Abstract: Annual Meeting of the American Philological Society 2009

3 Foxcroft, Louise, *Hot Flushes, Cold Science: A history of the modern menopause*, Granta Books, London 2009

This meticulously researched and entertaining book traces the history of 'the change of life' from its appearance in classical texts, to the medical literatures of the 18th century, to up-to-the-minute contemporary clinical approaches.

4 Foxcroft, Louise, *Hot Flushes, Cold Science: A history of the modern menopause*, Granta Books, London 2009

5 Bremmer J. in *Sexual Asymmetry: Studies in Ancient Society: The old women of ancient Greece*, (Editors) J Block, P Mason; Amsterdam: JC Gieben pp191–215

6 Foxcroft, Louise, *Hot Flushes, Cold Science: A history of the modern menopause*, Granta Books, London 2009

7 Foxcroft, Louise, *Hot Flushes, Cold Science: A history of the modern menopause*, Granta Books, London 2009

CHAPTER 2 The anatomy and physiology of the menopause

8 Prometrium Research, data submitted to FDA 1998 from the *Merck Manual*, 17th Edition, Whitehouse Station, Merck Research Laboratories 1999

9 Diczfalusy E, 'Estetrol: vita nova for a fetal steroid', *Climacteric*; 2008 Suppl.1. vol.11:1–599

10 Marker R, 'The Marker Degradation', Described in National Historic Chemical Landmarks, www.en.wikipedia.org/wiki/Marker_degradation. Accessed Jan 2010

11 Wren BG, McFarland K, Edwards L, et al, 'Effect of transdermal progesterone cream on endometrium, bleeding pattern and plasma progesterone levels in postmenopausal women', *Climacteric* 2000; 3:155–160

12 Wren BG, Champion SM, Zoa Manga R, Eden JA, 'Transdermal progesterone and its effect on vasomotor symptoms, blood lipid levels, bone metabolic markers, moods and quality of life for postmenopausal women', *Menopause* 2003; 10:13–18

13 Benster B, Carey A, Wadsworth F, et al, 'A double-blind placebo controlled study to evaluate the effect of progestelle progesterone cream on post-menopausal women', *Menopause Int.* 2009; 15:63–69

14 Royal College of General Practitioners Oral Contraceptive Study, *BMJ* 2010;340:927

15 Wilson R, *Feminine Forever*, WW Allen, London 1966

16 Lindsay R, Hart DM, Aitken JM, et al, 'Long term prevention of post menopausal osteoporosis by oestrogen', *Lancet* 1976;1:1038–39

Inderjeeth CA, Foo ACH, Lai MYA, Glendenning P, 'Efficacy and safety of pharmacological agents in managing osteoporosis in the old: Review of the evidence, *Bone* 2009;44:744–751

17 Rossouw JE, Prentice RL, Manson JE, et al, 'Hormone therapy may be safer in younger women? A best evidence review', *JAMA* 2007; 297:1465–1477

Nachtigall LE, Nachtigall RH, Nachtigall RD, Beckman EM, 'Estrogen replacement therapy II : A prospective of the relationship to carcinoma and cardiovascular and metabolic problems', *Obstet. Gynecol.* 1979; 54:74–9

Penotti M, Nencioni T, Gabrielli L, et al, 'Blood flow variations in internal carotid and middle cerebral arteries induced by postmenopausal hormone replacement therapy', *Am J Obstet Gynecol* 1993; 169:1226-32
Mosca L, 'The role of hormone replacement therapy in the prevention of postmenopausal heart disease', *Arch. Intern. Med.* 2000; 160:2263–2272
18 Yaffe K, 'Hormone therapy and the brain', *Editorial JAMA* 2003; 289:2717–18
19 Paganini-Hill A, Corrada MM, Kawas CH, 'Increased longevity in older users of postmenopausal estrogen therapy: The Leisure World Cohort Study', *Menopause J. Nth. Am. Menop. Society* 2006; 13:12–18
20 Hulley S, Grady D, Bush T, et al, 'Randomized trial of estrogen plus progestin for secondary prevention of coronary heart disease in postmenopausal women: Heart and Estrogen/progestin Replacement Study (HERS) Research Group', *JAMA* 2002; 288:321–333
21 Burger H.G., *The Menopause Transition,* The Menopause: Key issues, Bailliere's Clinical Obstetrics and Gynaecology, Ed. D. Barlow, London 1996.
22 Cass V, *The Elusive Orgasm*, Rockpool Publishing, Dulwich Hill , NSW, Australia, 2007

CHAPTER 3 The women's health initiative study

23 Rossouw JE, Anderson GL, Prentice RL, et al, 'Risks and benefits of estrogen plus progestin in healthy postmenopausal women: principal results from the Women's Health Initiative randomized controlled trial', *JAMA* 2002; 288:321–333
24 Swallen K, 'Newspaper coverage of the 1988 aspirin and the 2002 hormone therapy randomized clinical trials', University of Wisconsin—Madison CDE Working Paper No. 2003–06
25 Tattersall M, 'Risks and benefits of postmenopausal combined hormone replacement therapy', *Editorial MJA* 2002; 177:173–174
26 Beral V for the Million Women Study Collaborators: 'Breast cancer and hormone replacement therapy in the Million Women Study', *Lancet* 2003; 362:419–27
27 Shapiro S, 'The million women study: potential biases do not allow uncritical acceptance of the data', *Climacteric* 2004; 7:3–7.
28 Shapiro S, 'The million women study: potential biases do not allow uncritical acceptance of the data', *Climacteric* 2004; 7:3–7.
Burger H, 'Another look at WHI and its implications for hormone therapy', *Changes* 2006; 2:4–77
Bluming AZ, 'Hormone replacement therapy: The debate should continue', *Geriatrics*; 2004;59:30–37
Speroff L, 'The million women study and breast cancer', *Maturitas* 2003; 46:1–6
29 Rossouw JE, Anderson GL, Prentice RL, et al, 'Risks and benefits of estrogen plus progestin in healthy postmenopausal women: principal results from the Women's Health Initiative randomized controlled trial', *JAMA* 2002; 288:321–333
30 Anderson GL for the writing group for the Women's Health Initiative Investigators: 'Effects of conjugated equine estrogen in postmenopausal women with hysterectomy', *JAMA* 2004; 291:1701–1712

31 LaCroix AZ, Chlebowski RT, Manson JE, et al, 'Health outcomes after stopping conjugated estrogen among postmenopausal women with a prior hysterectomy', *JAMA* 2011; 305:1305–14

32 Burger H, 'Another look at WHI and its implications for hormone therapy', *Changes* 2006; 2:4–7

33 Bluming AZ, 'Hormone replacement therapy: The debate should continue', *Geriatrics*; 2004;59:30–37

34 Pines A, Personal comment in *IMS* newsletter, January 2010

35 Pines A, Sturdee DW, MacLennan AH et al, 'The heart of the WHI Study: time for hormone therapy policies to be revised', *Climacteric* 2007; 10:267–269

36 Karim R, Dell RM, Greene DF, et al, 'Hip fracture in postmenopausal women after cessation of hormone therapy: results from a prospective study in a large health management organisation', *Menopause*, 2011;18:1172–1177

37 MacLennan A, MacLennan A, 'Menopause: Presenting a positive outlook', published by the Australian Menopause Society 2011

38 Rossouw JE, Prentice RL, Manson JE, et al, 'Hormone therapy may be safer in younger women? A best evidence review', *JAMA* 2007; 297:1465–1477
Anderson GL for the writing group for the Women's Health Initiative Investigators: 'Effects of conjugated equine estrogen in postmenopausal women with hysterectomy', *JAMA* 2004; 291:1701–1712

39 Bluming AZ, Tavris C, 'Hormone replacement therapy. Real concerns and false alarms', *Cancer J.* 2009; 15:93–104
Stram DO, Liu Y, Henderson KD, et al, 'Age-specific effects of hormone therapy on overall mortality and ischaemic heart disease mortality among women in the California Teachers study Menopause', 2011;18:253–261
Hershman DL, Shao TH, Kushi L et al. 'Effect of early discontinuation or non-adherence to adjuvant therapy on mortality in women with breast cancer; *J Clin Oncol* 2010;28:15
Paganini-Hill A, Corrada MM, Kawas CH, 'Increased longevity in older users of postmenopausal estrogen therapy: The Leisure World Cohort Study', *Menopause J. Nth. Am. Menop. Society* 2006; 13:12–18

SECTION TWO: MENOPAUSE AND HEALTH

CHAPTER 4 Hormones and genital cancers

40 Ziel HK, Finkle WD,'Increased risk of endometrial carcinoma among users of conjugated estrogens', *N. Engl. J. Med.* 1975; 293:1167–70
Smith DC, Prentice R, Thompson DJ, Herman WL, 'Association of exogenous estrogens and endometrial cancer', *N. Engl. J. Med.* 975; 293:1164–1168
Mack TM, Pike MC, Henderson BE, et al Estrogens and endometrial cancer in a retirement community, *N. Engl. J. Med.* 1976; 294:1262–1267
Pickar JH, 'The endometrium—from estrogens alone to TSECS', *Climacteric* 2009; 12:463–477

41 Pickar JH, 'The endometrium—from estrogens alone to TSECS', *Climacteric* 2009; 12:463–477

42 Beral V for the Million Women Study Collaborators: 'Ovarian cancer and hormone replacement therapy in the Million Women Study', *Lancet* 2007; 369(9574):1703–1

43 Rodriguez C, Patel AV, Calle, et al, 'Estrogen replacement therapy and ovarian cancer mortality', *JAMA* 2001; 285:1460–1465

44 Shapiro S, 'False alarm: postmenopausal hormone therapy and ovarian cancer', *Climacteric* 2007; 10:466–470

45 The Lancet Editors, 'The case for preventing ovarian cancer', *Lancet* 2008: 371:275

46 Rossouw JE, Anderson GL, Prentice RL, et al, 'Risks and benefits of estrogen plus progestin in healthy postmenopausal women: principal results from the Women's Health Initiative randomized controlled trial', *JAMA* 2002; 288:321–333

47 Beral V for the Million Women Study Collaborators: 'Ovarian cancer and hormone replacement therapy in the Million Women Study', *Lancet* 2007; 369(9574):1703–10

48 Welch HG, Woloshin S, Schwartz LM, 'The sea of uncertainty surrounding ductal carcinoma in situ—the price of screening mammography', *Editorial J. Nat. Cancer Inst.* 2008; 100(4): 228–9
Esserman L, Shieh Y, Thompson L, 'Rethinking screening for breast and prostate cancer', *JAMA* 2009; 302:1685–9

49 Welch HG, Woloshin S, Schwartz LM, 'The sea of uncertainty surrounding ductal carcinoma in situ—the price of screening mammography', *Editorial J. Nat. Cancer Inst.* 2008; 100(4): 228–9
Esserman L, Shieh Y, Thompson L, 'Rethinking screening for breast and prostate cancer', *JAMA* 2009; 302:1685–92
Jorgensen KJ, Gotzsche PC, 'Overdiagnosis in publicly organized mammographic screening programmes: a systematic review of incidence trends', The Nordic Cochrane Centre, Rigshospitalet Dept. 3343, *Blegdamsvej* 9. DK-2100 Copenhagen
Tabar L, Vitak B, Chen T, 'Swedish two-county trial: impact of mammographic screening on breast cancer mortality during three decades', *Radiology* 2011. Paper available prior to publication in Epub

50 Tabar L, Vitak B, Chen T, 'Swedish two-county trial: impact of mammographic screening on breast cancer mortality during three decades', *Radiology* 2011. Paper available prior to publication in Epub

51 Jorgensen KJ, Gotzsche PC, 'Overdiagnosis in publicly organized mammographic screening programmes: a systematic review of incidence trends', The Nordic Cochrane Centre, Rigshospitalet Dept. 3343, *Blegdamsvej* 9. DK-2100 Copenhagen

52 Seigneurin A, Francois O, Labarere J, et al. Overdiagnosis from non-progressive cancer detected by screening mammography: stochastic simulation study with calibration to population based registry data, BMJ 2011;343:701-7

53 Shapiro S, Farmer RDT, Stevenson J, et al, 'Does hormone replacement therapy cause breast cancer? An application of causal principles to three studies', *Family Planning* (2011).doi: 1136/jfprhc-2011-100229
Wren BG, 'The origin of breast cancer', *Menopause* 2007;14:1060–1068

54 Shapiro S, Farmer RDT, Stevenson J, et al, 'Does hormone replacement therapy cause breast cancer? An application of causal principles to three studies', *Family Planning* (2011).doi: 1136/jfprhc-2011-100229

55 Welch HG, Woloshin S, Schwartz LM, 'The sea of uncertainty surrounding ductal carcinoma in situ - the price of screening mammography', *Editorial J. Nat. Cancer Inst.* 2008; 100(4): 228–9
Esserman L, Shieh Y, Thompson L, 'Rethinking screening for breast and prostate cancer', *JAMA* 2009; 302:1685–92
Wren BG, 'The origin of breast cancer', *Menopause* 2007;14:1060–1068
56 Welch HG, Woloshin S, Schwartz LM, 'The sea of uncertainty surrounding ductal carcinoma in situ - the price of screening mammography', *Editorial J. Nat. Cancer Inst.* 2008; 100(4): 228–9
Esserman L, Shieh Y, Thompson L, 'Rethinking screening for breast and prostate cancer', *JAMA* 2009; 302:1685–92
Jorgensen KJ, Gotzsche PC, 'Overdiagnosis in publicly organized mammographic screening programmes: a systematic review of incidence trends', The Nordic Cochrane Centre, Rigshospitalet Dept. 3343, *Blegdamsvej* 9. DK-2100 Copenhagen
Nielsen M, Thomsen JL, Primdahl S, et al, 'Breast cancer and atypia among young and middle aged women: a study of 110 medico-legal autopsies', *Brit. J. Cancer* 1987; 56:814–819
Welch HG, Black WC, 'Using autopsy series to estimate the disease reservoir for ductal carcinoma in situ of the breast', *Ann. Int. Med.* 1997;127:1023–1028
57 Jorgensen KJ, Gotzsche PC, 'Overdiagnosis in publicly organized mammographic screening programmes: a systematic review of incidence trends', The Nordic Cochrane Centre, Rigshospitalet Dept. 3343, *Blegdamsvej* 9. DK-2100 Copenhagen
58 Nielsen M, Thomsen JL, Primdahl S, et al, 'Breast cancer and atypia among young and middle aged women: a study of 110 medico-legal autopsies', *Brit. J. Cancer* 1987; 56:814–819
Welch HG, Black WC, 'Using autopsy series to estimate the disease reservoir for ductal carcinoma in situ of the breast', *Ann. Int. Med.* 1997;127:1023–1028
Bhathal PS, Brown RW, Lesueur GC, Russell IS, 'Frequency of benign and malignant breast lesions in 207 consecutive autopsies in Australian women', *Br. J. Cancer*, 1985; 51: 271–278
Alpers CE, Wellington SR, 'The prevalence of carcinoma in-situ in normal and cancer associated breasts', *Human Pathol.* 1985;16:796–807
59 Nielsen M, Thomsen JL, Primdahl S, et al, 'Breast cancer and atypia among young and middle aged women: a study of 110 medico-legal autopsies', *Brit. J. Cancer* 1987; 56:814–819
Bhathal PS, Brown RW, Lesueur GC, Russell IS, 'Frequency of benign and malignant breast lesions in 207 consecutive autopsies in Australian women', *Br. J. Cancer*, 1985; 51: 271–278
Alpers CE, Wellington SR, 'The prevalence of carcinoma in-situ in normal and cancer associated breasts', *Human Pathol.* 1985;16:796–807
60 Nielsen M, Thomsen JL, Primdahl S, et al, 'Breast cancer and atypia among young and middle aged women: a study of 110 medico-legal autopsies', *Brit. J. Cancer* 1987; 56:814–819
Welch HG, Black WC, 'Using autopsy series to estimate the disease reservoir for ductal carcinoma in situ of the breast', *Ann. Int. Med.* 1997;127:1023–1028

Bartow SW, Pathak DR, Black WC, et al, 'Prevalence of benign, atypical, and malignant breast lesions in populations at different risk for breast cancer: A forensic autopsy study', *Cancer* 1987;60:2751–2760

Bhathal PS, Brown RW, Lesueur GC, Russell IS, 'Frequency of benign and malignant breast lesions in 207 consecutive autopsies in Australian women', *Br J Cancer*, 1985; 51: 271-278

Feur EJ, Wun LM, 'Probability of developing or dying of breast cancer', *DEVCAN—Nat. Cancer Inst.* 1999 Available at: http://imaginis.com./breasthealth/statistics.asp

61 Rossouw JE, Anderson GL, Prentice RL, et al, 'Risks and benefits of estrogen plus progestin in healthy postmenopausal women: principal results from the Women's Health Initiative randomized controlled trial', *JAMA* 2002; 288:321–333

Welch HG, Woloshin S, Schwartz LM, 'The sea of uncertainty surrounding ductal carcinoma in situ - the price of screening mammography', *Editorial J. Nat. Cancer Inst.* 2008; 100(4): 228–9

Esserman L, Shieh Y, Thompson L, 'Rethinking screening for breast and prostate cancer', *JAMA* 2009; 302:1685–92

Wren BG, 'The origin of breast cancer', *Menopause* 2007;14:1060–1068

Nielsen M, Thomsen JL, Primdahl S, et al, 'Breast cancer and atypia among young and middle aged women: a study of 110 medico-legal autopsies', *Brit. J. Cancer* 1987; 56:814–819

Welch HG, Black WC, 'Using autopsy series to estimate the disease reservoir for ductal carcinoma in situ of the breast', *Ann. Int. Med.* 1997;127:1023–1028

Bartow SW, Pathak DR, Black WC, et al, 'Prevalence of benign, atypical, and malignant breast lesions in populations at different risk for breast cancer: A forensic autopsy study', *Cancer* 1987;60:2751–2760

Bhathal PS, Brown RW, Lesueur GC, Russell IS, 'Frequency of benign and malignant breast lesions in 207 consecutive autopsies in Australian women', *Br. J. Cancer*, 1985; 51: 271–278

Alpers CE, Wellington SR, 'The prevalence of carcinoma in-situ in normal and cancer associated breasts', *Human Pathol.* 1985;16:796–807

62 Feur EJ, Wun LM *Probability of developing or dying of breast cancer* DEVCAN—Nat Cancer Inst, 1999 Available at: http://imaginis.com./breasthealth/statistics.asp

63 Bluming AZ, Tavris C, 'Hormone replacement therapy. Real concerns and false alarms', *Cancer J.* 2009; 15:93–104

64 Bluming AZ, Tavris C, 'Hormone replacement therapy. Real concerns and false alarms', *Cancer J.* 2009; 15:93–104

65 Ong EK, Glantz SA, 'Constructing sound science and good epidemiology', *Am. J. Publ. Health* 2001; 91:1749–1757

66 Holland JF, Pogo BGT, 'Mouse mammary tumor virus-like viral infection and human breast cancer', *Clin. Cancer Res.* 2004; 10:5647–50

CHAPTER 5 Estrogen and the cardiovascular system

67 Clarkson T, Appt S, 'Controversies about HRT: lessons from monkey models', *Maturitas* 2005; 51:64–74

Lobo RA, 'Postmenopausal hormones and coronary artery disease: potential benefits and risks', *Climacteric* 2007; 10 Suppl. 2:21–26
Merz CN, Johnson BD, Berga SL, et al, 'Total estrogen time and obstructive coronary disease in women: insights from the NHLBI-sponsored Women's Ischaemia Syndrome Evaluation (WISE)', *J. Women's Health* 2009; 18:1315–22
Ingelsson E, Lundholm C, Johansson ALV, Altman D, 'Hysterectomy and risk of cardiovascular disease in a population based cohort study', *Europ. Heart J.* 2011; 32:745–750
Sullivan JM, 'Estrogen replacement therapy', *Am. J. Med.* 1996;101:56S–59S
Herrington DM, Werbel BL, Riley WA, et al, 'Individual and combined effects of estrogen/progestin therapy and lovastatin on lipids and flow mediated vasodilatation in postmenopausal women with coronary artery disease', *J. Am. Coll. Cardiology* 1999;33:2030–2037

68 Ingelsson E, Lundholm C, Johansson ALV, Altman D *Hysterectomy and risk of cardiovascular disease in a population based cohort study.* Europ. Heart J 2011;32:745-750

69 Clarkson T, Appt S, 'Controversies about HRT: lessons from monkey models', *Maturitas* 2005; 51:64–74

70 Penotti M, Nencioni T, Gabrielli L, et al, 'Blood flow variations in internal carotid and middle cerebral arteries induced by postmenopausal hormone replacement therapy', *Am J Obstet Gynecol* 1993; 169:1226-32
Mosca L, 'The role of hormone replacement therapy in the prevention of postmenopausal heart disease', *Arch. Intern. Med.* 2000; 160:2263–2272
Hulley S, Grady D, Bush T, et al, 'Randomized trial of estrogen plus progestin for secondary prevention of coronary heart disease in postmenopausal women: Heart and Estrogen/progestin Replacement Study (HERS) Research Group', *JAMA* 1998; 280:605–613
Lobo RA, 'Postmenopausal hormones and coronary artery disease: potential benefits and risks', *Climacteric* 2007; 10 Suppl. 2:21–26
Merz CN, Johnson BD, Berga SL, et al, 'Total estrogen time and obstructive coronary disease in women: insights from the NHLBI-sponsored Women's Ischaemia Syndrome Evaluation (WISE)', *J. Women's Health* 2009; 18:1315–22
Herrington DM, Werbel BL, Riley WA, et al, 'Individual and combined effects of estrogen/progestin therapy and lovastatin on lipids and flow mediated vasodilatation in postmenopausal women with coronary artery disease', *J. Am. Coll. Cardiology* 1999;33:2030–2037
Grodstein D, Manson JE, Colditz GA, et al, 'A prospective, observational study of postmenopausal hormone therapy and primary prevention of cardiovascular disease', *Ann. Intern. Med.* 2000; 133:933–941

71 Sullivan JM, 'Estrogen replacement therapy', *Am. J. Med.* 1996;101:56S–59
Herrington DM, Werbel BL, Riley WA, et al, 'Individual and combined effects of estrogen/progestin therapy and lovastatin on lipids and flow mediated vasodilatation in postmenopausal women with coronary artery disease', *J. Am. Coll. Cardiology* 1999;33:2030–2037

Manson JE, Allison MA, Rossouw JE, et al, 'Estrogen therapy and coronary artery calcification', *N. Engl. J. Med.* 2007; 356:2591–2602

Shufelt CL, Bairey Merz CN, 'Contraceptive hormone use and cardiovascular disease', J. Am. Coll. Cardiol. 2009;53:221–231

Lakoski S, Brosnihan B, Herrington DM, 'Hormone therapy, C-Reactive protein and progression of atherosclerosis: Data from the estrogen replacement on progression of coronary artery atherosclerosis trial', *Am. Heart J.* 2005;150:907–911

Lieberman EH, Gerhard M, Uehatu A, et al, 'Estrogen improves endothelial dependent flow mediated vasodilatation in post-menopausal women', *Ann. Int. Med.* 1994;121:936–941

Schindler TH, Campis R, Dorsey D, et al, 'Effect of hormone replacement therapy on vasomotor function of coronary micro-circulation in postmenopausal women with medically treated cardiovascular risk factors', *Eur. Heart J.* 2009;30:978–986

72 Mosca L, 'The role of hormone replacement therapy in the prevention of postmenopausal heart disease', *Arch. Intern. Med.* 2000; 160:2263–2272

Lieberman EH, Gerhard M, Uehatu A, et al, 'Estrogen improves endothelial dependent flow mediated vasodilatation in post-menopausal women', *Ann. Int. Med.* 1994;121:936–941

Schindler TH, Campis R, Dorsey D, et al, 'Effect of hormone replacement therapy on vasomotor function of coronary micro-circulation in postmenopausal women with medically treated cardiovascular risk factors', *Eur. Heart J.* 2009;30:978–986

73 Canonico M, Plu-Bureau G, Lowe GDO, Scarabin P-L, 'Hormone replacement therapy and risk of thromboembolism in postmenopausal women: A systematic review and meta analysis', *BMJ* 2008; 336:1227–30

Scarabin P-Y, Oger E, Plu-Bureau G, 'Differential association of oral and transdermal oestrogen-replacement therapy with venous thromboembolism risk', *The Lancet* 2003; 362:428–32

74 Clarkson T, Appt S, 'Controversies about HRT: lessons from monkey models', *Maturitas* 2005; 51:64–74

75 Mosca L, 'The role of hormone replacement therapy in the prevention of postmenopausal heart disease', *Arch. Intern. Med.* 2000; 160:2263–2272

76 Herrington DM, Werbel BL, Riley WA, et al, 'Individual and combined effects of estrogen/progestin therapy and lovastatin on lipids and flow mediated vasodilatation in postmenopausal women with coronary artery disease', *J. Am. Coll. Cardiology* 1999;33:2030–2037

Manson JE, Allison MA, Rossouw JE, et al, 'Estrogen therapy and coronary artery calcification', *N. Engl. J. Med.* 2007; 356:2591–2602

Lieberman EH, Gerhard M, Uehatu A, et al, 'Estrogen improves endothelial dependent flow mediated vasodilatation in post-menopausal women', *Ann. Int. Med.* 1994;121:936–941

Herrington DM, Werbel BL, Riley WA, et al, 'Individual and combined effects of estrogen/progestin therapy and lovastatin on lipids and flow mediated vasodilatation in postmenopausal women with coronary artery disease', *J. Am. Coll. Cardiology* 1999;33:2030–2037

Manson JE, Allison MA, Rossouw JE, et al, 'Estrogen therapy and coronary artery calcification', *N. Engl. J. Med.* 2007; 356:2591–2602
Lieberman EH, Gerhard M, Uehatu A, et al, 'Estrogen improves endothelial dependent flow mediated vasodilatation in post-menopausal women', *Ann. Int. Med.* 1994;121:936–941
Schindler TH, Campis R, Dorsey D, et al, 'Effect of hormone replacement therapy on vasomotor function of coronary micro-circulation in postmenopausal women with medically treated cardiovascular risk factors', *Eur. Heart J.* 2009;30:978–986

77 Hulley S, Grady D, Bush T, et al, 'Randomized trial of estrogen plus progestin for secondary prevention of coronary heart disease in postmenopausal women: Heart and Estrogen/progestin Replacement Study (HERS) Research Group', *JAMA* 1998; 280:605–613

78 Rossouw JE, Anderson GL, Prentice RL, et al, 'Risks and benefits of estrogen plus progestin in healthy postmenopausal women: principal results from the Women's Health Initiative randomized controlled trial', *JAMA* 2002; 288:321–333

79 Schierbeck LL, Rejnmark L, Tofteng CL, et al 'Effect of hormone replacement therapy on cardiovascular events in recently menopausal women; randomised trial', *BMJ*, 2012;345: e609.

80 Canonico M, Plu-Bureau G, Lowe GDO, Scarabin P-L, 'Hormone replacement therapy and risk of thromboembolism in postmenopausal women: A systematic review and meta analysis', *BMJ* 2008; 336:1227–30
Scarabin P-Y, Oger E, Plu-Bureau G, 'Differential association of oral and transdermal oestrogen-replacement therapy with venous thromboembolism risk', *The Lancet* 2003; 362:428–32

81 Manson JE, Allison MA, Rossouw JE, et al, 'Estrogen therapy and coronary artery calcification', *N. Engl. J. Med.* 2007; 356:2591–2602

CHAPTER 6 Osteopaenia and osteoporosis

82 Seeman E, Delmas P, 'Bone quality: The material and structural basis of bone strength and fragility', *New Engl. J. Med.* 2006; 354:2250–2259

83 Karim R, Dell RM, Greene DF, et al, 'Hip fracture in postmenopausal women after cessation of hormone therapy: results from a prospective study in a large health management organisation', *Menopause*, 2011;18:1172–1177

CHAPTER 7 Hormones, brain function, memory and dementia

84 Australian Bureau of Statistics, 2011 'Causes of death, Australia, 2009', Cat. No.3303.0, Australian Bureau of Statistics, Canberra, viewed 30 July 2012, http://www.abs.gov.au/Causes of Death, Australia,2009

85 Ott A, Breteler MM, vanHarskamp F, et al, 'Incidence and risk of dementia: the Rotterdam study', *Am. J. Epidemiol.* 1998;147:574–580

86 Whitmer RA, Quesenberry CP, Zhou J, Yaffe K, 'Timing of hormone therapy and dementia. The critical window theory revisited', *Ann. Neurology* 2011; 69:163–69

87 Csoreigh L, Andersson E, Fried G, 'Transcriptional analysis of estrogen effects in human embryonic neurons and glial cells', *Neuroendocrinology* 2009;89:171–178

Cole SL, Vassar R, 'The Alzheimers disease - secretase enzyme, BACE1', *Molecular Neurodegeneration* 2007;2:2
Behl C, 'Estrogen, mystery drug for the brain? The neuroprotective effect of the female sex hormone', 2001, Springer NY pp116–166
88 Ott A, Breteler MM, van Harskamp F, et al, 'Incidence and risk of dementia: the Rotterdam study', *Am. J. Epidemiol.* 1998;147:574–580
89 Csoreigh L, Andersson E, Fried G, 'Transcriptional analysis of estrogen effects in human embryonic neurons and glial cells', *Neuroendocrinology* 2009;89:171–178
Cole SL, Vassar R, 'The Alzheimers disease -secretase enzyme, BACE1', *Molecular Neurodegeneration* 2007;2:2
Behl C, 'Estrogen, mystery drug for the brain? The neuroprotective effect of the female sex hormone', 2001, Springer NY pp116–166
90 Wren BG, 2004, *Understanding Menopause and Hormonal Therapy*, 2nd edition, McGraw-Hill, North Ryde
91 Ettinger B, Friedman GD, Bush T, Queensberry CP, 'Reduced mortality associated with long-term postmenopausal estrogen therapy', *Obstet. Gynecol.* 1996;87:6–12
Visvanathan K, Chlebowski RT, Hurley P, et al, 'American Society of Clinical Oncology clinical practice guideline update on the use of pharmacologic interventions including Tamoxifen, Raloxifene and aromatase inhibition for breast cancer risk reduction', *J. Clin. Oncol.* 2009; 27:3235–3258

SECTION THREE: MANAGEMENT OF MENOPAUSE

CHAPTER 9 Hormone replacement therapy regimens

92 Ziel HK, Finkle WD, 'Increased risk of endometrial carcinoma among users of conjugated estrogens', *N. Engl. J. Med.* 1975; 293:1167–70
Smith DC, Prentice R, Thompson DJ, Herman WL, 'Association of exogenous estrogens and endometrial cancer', *N. Engl. J. Med.* 975; 293:1164–1168
Mack TM, Pike MC, Henderson BE, et al Estrogens and endometrial cancer in a retirement community, *N. Engl. J. Med.* 1976; 294:1262–1267
93 Hulley S, Grady D, Bush T, et al, 'Randomized trial of estrogen plus progestin for secondary prevention of coronary heart disease in postmenopausal women: Heart and Estrogen/progestin Replacement Study (HERS) Research Group', *JAMA* 1998; 280:605–613
94 Wren BG, Day RO, McLaughlan AJ, Williams KM, 'Pharmacokinetics of estradiol, progesterone, testosterone and dehydroepiandrosterone after transbuccal administration to postmenopausal women', *Climacteric*, 2003; 6:104–111
95 Wren BG, 2004, *Understanding Menopause and Hormonal Therapy*, 2nd edition, McGraw-Hill, North Ryde
96 NAMS, 'Updated position statement on estrogen and progestogen', *Menopause* 2010; 17:242–255
97 Stram DO, Henderson KD, Sullivan-Halley J, et al, 'Age-specific effects of hormone therapy on overall mortality and ischaemic heart disease mortality among women in the California Teachers Study', *Menopause* 2011;18:253-261

98 Hershman DL, Shao TH, Kushi L et al, 'Effect of early discontinuation or non-adherence to adjuvant therapy on mortality in women with breast cancer', *J Clin Oncol 2010*;28:15

99 Salpeter S, Cheng J, Thabane L, et al, 'Bayesian meta-analysis of hormone therapy and mortality in younger postmenopausal women', *Am J Med.* 2009:122;1016-1022

100 Paganini-Hill A, Corrada MM, Kawas CH, 'Increased longevity in older users of postmenopausal estrogen therapy: The Leisure World Cohort Study', *Menopause J. Nth. Am. Menop. Society 2006; 13:12–18*

101 Ettinger B, Friedman GD, Bush T, Queensberry CP, 'Reduced mortality associated with long-term postmenopausal estrogen therapy', *Obstet. Gynecol.* 1996;87:6–12

CHAPTER 10 Methods of delivering HRT regimens

102 Wren BG, Day RO, McLaughlan AJ, Williams KM, 'Pharmacokinetics of estradiol, progesterone, testosterone and dehydroepiandrosterone after transbuccal administration to postmenopausal women', *Climacteric*, 2003; 6:104–111.

(Biochemical measures of hormones can be confusing if it is not realised that estradiol in blood is measured in picomol/litre (pmol./L) while progesterone and testosterone are measured in nanomol/litre (nmol/L). (1nmol = 1000pmol). The amount of estradiol that is necessary to control post-menopausal symptoms is relatively small (150–500pmol/L), whereas the amount of progesterone necessary to produce a secretory change or to prevent endometrial growth is relatively large – 10,000–50,000pmol/L (10–50nmol/L).

CHAPTER 12 Other medical treatments for the menopause

103 Visvanathan K, Chlebowski RT, Hurley P, et al, 'American Society of Clinical Oncology clinical practice guideline update on the use of pharmacologic interventions including Tamoxifen, Raloxifene and aromatase inhibition for breast cancer risk reduction', *J. Clin. Oncol.* 2009; 27:3235–3258

Vogel VG, Constantino JP, Wickerham DL et al, 'Effects of tamoxifen vs raloxifene on the risk of developing invasive breast cancer and other disease outcomes: the NSABP Study of Tamoxifen and Raloxifene (STAR) P–2 trial', *JAMA* 2006; 295:2727–2741

Cummings SR, Ettinger B, Delmas PD, et al, 'The effects of tibolone in older post-menopausal women', *New Engl. J. Med.* 2008; 359:697–708

Lewiecki EM, 'Bazedoxifene and bazedoxifene combined with conjugated estrogens for the management of postmenopausal osteoporosis', *Expert Opin. Investig. Drugs*, 2007; 16:1663–1672

104 Lewiecki EM, 'Bazedoxifene and bazedoxifene combined with conjugated estrogens for the management of postmenopausal osteoporosis', *Expert Opin. Investig. Drugs*, 2007; 16:1663–1672

CHAPTER 13 Complementary medicine and alternative therapies for menopause

105 Newton KM, 'The use of alternative therapies for menopausal symptoms', *Obstet. Gynecol.*, 2002;100:18–25

106 Ernst E, 'Obstacles to research in complementary and alternative medicine', Editorial *MJA*, 2003;179:279–280

107 Thomas KJ, Nicholl JP, Coleman P. *Use and expenditure on complementary medicine in England: a population based survey*. Complementary Therapies in Medicine 2001;9:2-11

108 Rossouw JE, Anderson GL, Prentice RL, et al, 'Risks and benefits of estrogen plus progestin in healthy postmenopausal women: principal results from the Women's Health Initiative randomized controlled trial', *JAMA* 2002; 288:321–333

109 Prometrium Research, data submitted to FDA 1998 from the *Merck Manual*, 17th Edition, Whitehouse Station, Merck Research Laboratories 1999

110 'Hepatoxicity with black cohosh', *Australian Adverse Drug Reaction Bulletin*, Vol. 25, No. 2

111 Whiting PW, Clouston A, Kerlin P, 'Black cohosh and herbal remedies associated with acute hepatitis', *MJA*, 2000;1777:440–443

112 Blackwell R, 'Adverse events involving certain Chinese Herbal Medicines and the response of the profession',*Journal Chinese Medicine* 1996, accessed 13.01.2012 http;//www.jcm.co.uk/media/sample-articles/50–12.pdf

113 Wren BG, McFarland K, Edwards L, et al, 'Effect of transdermal progesterone cream on endometrium, bleeding pattern and plasma progesterone levels in postmenopausal women', *Climacteric* 2000; 3:155–160

Benster B, Carey A, Wadsworth F, et al, 'A double-blind placebo controlled study to evaluate the effect of progestelle progesterone cream on post-menopausal women', *Menopause Int.* 2009; 15:63–69

CHAPTER 14 Hormone therapy for a woman following breast cancer, endometriosis or fibroids

114 Welch HG, Woloshin S, Schwartz LM, 'The sea of uncertainty surrounding ductal carcinoma in-situ – the price of screening mammography', *Editorial J. Nat. Cancer Inst.* 2008; 100(4): 228–9

Esserman L, Shieh Y, Thompson L, 'Rethinking screening for breast and prostate cancer', *JAMA* 2009; 302:1685–92

Jorgensen KJ, Gotzsche PC, 'Overdiagnosis in publicly organized mammographic screening programmes: a systematic review of incidence trends', The Nordic Cochrane Centre, Rigshospitalet Dept. 3343, *Blegdamsvej* 9. DK-2100 Copenhagen

115 Vassilopoulou-Selin R, Zolinski C, 'Estrogen replacement therapy in women with breast cancer: a survey of patient attitudes', *Am. J. Med. Sci.*1992;304:145–149

116 Manson JE, 'Estrogen therapy, breast cancer, and heart disease', *Medscape* 28.04.2011 http://www.medscape.com/viewarticle/740960?src=mp&spon=16 accessed 08.05.2011

117 Dew J, Eden J, Beller E, et al, 'A cohort study of hormone replacement therapy given to women previously treated for breast cancer', *Climacteric* 1998;1:137–142

Dew J, Wren BG, Eden J, 'Tamoxifen, hormone receptors and hormone replacement therapy in women previously treated for breast cancer: a cohort study', *Climacteric* 2002; 5:151–155

Durna E, Wren BG, Heller, et al, 'Hormone replacement therapy after a diagnosis of breast cancer: cancer recurrence and mortality', *MJA* 2002;177:347–351

118 O'Meara ES, Rossing MA, Daling JR, et al, 'Hormone replacement therapy after a diagnosis of breast cancer in relation to recurrence and mortality', *J. Natl. Cancer Inst.* 2001;93:754–762

119 Royal College of Obstetricians and Gynaecologists, 'Pregnancy and breast cancer guideline', No.12;2004

SECTION FOUR: CHOICES

CHAPTER 15 The balance and beauty of ageing

120 Austad SN, 1997, *Why do we age?—What science is discovering about the body's journey through life.* John Wiley and Sons, Inc. New York

121 Austad SN *Why do we age?—What science is discovering about the body's journey through life.* John Wiley and Sons, Inc. New York 1997.
Steven Austad's very readable book investigates the history, the theories, and the personalities behind the quest to understand the nature of aging. It provides hard evidence from the front lines of research that science is closing in on the fundamental processes of human biology and life.

Menopause today

122 Reginster JY, Seeman E, DeVernejoul MC, et al, 'Strontium ranelate reduces the risk of non-vertebral fractures in post menopausal women with osteoporosis : TROPOS study', *J. Clin. Endocrinol Metab.* 2005; 90:2816–2822

123 Paganini-Hill A, Corrada MM, Kawas CH, 'Increased longevity in older users of postmenopausal estrogen therapy: The Leisure World Cohort Study', *Menopause J. Nth. Am. Menop.* Society 2006; 13:12–18

APPENDICES

APPENDIX 2 Oral hormone preparations: estrogen/progesterone

124 Kenemans P, Bundred NJ, Foidart J-M, et al, 'Safety and efficacy of tibolone in breast cancer patients with vaso-motor symptoms: a double blind, randomized, non-inferiority trial', *The Lancet* 2009; 10:135–146

125 Meunier PJ, Roux C, Seeman E, et al, 'The effect of strontium ranelate on the risk of vertebral fractures in women with post menopausal osteoporosis', *New Engl. J. Med.* 2004; 350:459–468

APPENDIX 5 SERMs

126 Visvanathan K, Chlebowski RT, Hurley P, et al, 'American Society of Clinical Oncology clinical practice guideline update on the use of pharmacologic interventions including Tamoxifen, Raloxifene and aromatase inhibition for breast cancer risk reduction', *J. Clin. Oncol.* 2009; 27:3235–3258
Vogel VG, Constantino JP, Wickerham DL et al, 'Effects of tamoxifen vs raloxifene on the risk of developing invasive breast cancer and other disease outcomes: the

NSABP Study of Tamoxifen and Raloxifene (STAR) P–2 trial', *JAMA* 2006; 295:2727–2741

127 Lewiecki EM, 'Bazedoxifene and bazedoxifene combined with conjugated estrogens for the management of postmenopausal osteoporosis', *Expert Opin. Investig. Drugs,* 2007; 16:1663–1672

APPENDIX 7 Treatment of osteopenia and osteoporosis

128 Reginster JY, Seeman E, DeVernejoul MC, et al, 'Strontium ranelate reduces the risk of non-vertebral fractures in post menopausal women with osteoporosis : TROPOS study', *J. Clin. Endocrinol Metab.* 2005 ;90:2816–2822
Sjoblom T, Jones S, Wood LD, et al, 'The consensus coding sequence of human breast and colorectal cancers', *Science* 2006; 314:268–274

APPENDIX 9 Hormones and cancer

129 Australian Bureau of Statistics, 2011, *Causes of death, Australia, 2009, cat.No.3303.*0, Australian Bureau of Statistics, Canberra, viewed 30 July, http://www.abs.gov.au/ Causes of Death, Australia, 2009

130 Hanahan D, Weinberg R, 'The hallmarks of cancer', *Cell,* 2000; 100:57–70
Perez-Losada J, Gonzalez-Sarmiento R *Breast cancer: a stem cell disease* Current Stem Cell Research and Therapy 2008; 3:55-65

131 Skinner M, 'Stem cells: insights into breast cancer heterogeneity', *Nature Rev. Cancer* 2010; 10:163–171
Perez-Losada J, Gonzalez-Sarmiento R 'Breast cancer: a stem cell disease', *Current Stem Cell Research and Therapy* 2008; 3:55-65

132 Skinner M, 'Stem cells: insights into breast cancer heterogeneity', *Nature Rev. Cancer* 2010; 10:163–171
Perez-Losada J, Gonzalez-Sarmiento R, 'Breast cancer: a stem cell disease', *Current Stem Cell Research and Therapy* 2008; 3:55–65
Steel M, 'Telomeres that shape our end', Commentary, *Lancet* 1995:345:935–936

133 Hanahan D, Weinberg R, 'The hallmarks of cancer', *Cell,* 2000; 100:57–70
Skinner M, 'Stem cells: insights into breast cancer heterogeneity', *Nature Rev. Cancer* 2010; 10:163–171
Steel M, 'Telomeres that shape our end', Commentary, *Lancet* 1995:345:935–936

134 Steel M, 'Telomeres that shape our end', Commentary, *Lancet* 1995:345:935–936

135 Hanahan D, Weinberg R, The hallmarks of cancer' *Cell,* 2000; 100:57–70
Skinner M, 'Stem cells: insights into breast cancer heterogeneity', *Nature Rev. Cancer* 2010; 10:163–171
Perez-Losada J, Gonzalez-Sarmiento R, 'Breast cancer: a stem cell disease', *Current Stem Cell Research and Therapy* 2008; 3:55–65
Steel M, 'Telomeres that shape our end', Commentary, *Lancet* 1995:345:935–936

136 Welch HG, Woloshin S, Schwartz LM, 'The sea of uncertainty surrounding ductal carcinoma in-situ – the price of screening mammography', *Editorial J. Nat. Cancer Inst.* 2008; 100(4): 228–9
Esserman L, Shieh Y, Thompson L, 'Rethinking screening for breast and prostate cancer', *JAMA* 2009; 302:1685–92

APPENDIX 10 Assessing research in medical studies

137 MacLennan A, MacLennan A, 'Menopause: Presenting a positive outlook', published by the Australian Menopause Society 2011

138 Rossouw JE, Anderson GL, Prentice RL, et al, 'Risks and benefits of estrogen plus progestin in healthy postmenopausal women: principal results from the Women's Health Initiative randomized controlled trial', *JAMA* 2002; 288:321–333
Beral V for the Million Women Study Collaborators: 'Breast cancer and hormone replacement therapy in the Million Women Study', *Lancet* 2003; 362:419–27

139 Anderson GL for the writing group for the Women's Health Initiative Investigators: 'Effects of conjugated equine estrogen in postmenopausal women with hysterectomy', *JAMA* 2004; 291:1701–1712

140 Nielsen M, Thomsen JL, Primdahl S, et al, 'Breast cancer and atypia among young and middle aged women: a study of 110 medico-legal autopsies', *Brit. J. Cancer* 1987; 56:814–819

141 Clarkson T, Appt S, 'Controversies about HRT: lessons from monkey models', *Maturitas* 2005; 51:64–74

142 Hanahan D, Weinberg R, 'The hallmarks of cancer', *Cell*, 2000; 100:57–70

143 Hulley S, Grady D, Bush T, et al, 'Randomized trial of estrogen plus progestin for secondary prevention of coronary heart disease in postmenopausal women: Heart and Estrogen/progestin Replacement Study (HERS) Research Group', *JAMA* 1998; 280:605–613

Acknowledgments

I would like to acknowledge the help and advice I have had from so many who have contributed to this book.

First, I would like to thank the women who, having read some of the books I had written for doctors, asked for a similar book, written specifically for women so they could understand and make their own decision about their need for hormone therapy. Then I would like to thank the many women who commented about their problems, their symptoms, their needs and their desires regarding their post-menopause, and who had requested that I address these issues. The content of the book is based on the comments and questions posed by them all.

In deciding to write this book I became aware of my own deficiency—I am not a woman! I could only guess at some of the feelings and concerns of a woman.

I deliberated about how to address this problem and in a stroke of pure good fortune decided to invite a friend and author to help me. Margaret Stephenson Meere was not only enthusiastic about the project, but has spent many hours as we debated the merits of a word, a sentence, a paragraph or the content of the many articles and items of information which we thought would be relevant to the content of the book. It was Margaret who introduced me to Lisa Hanrahan, our enthusiastic publisher at Rockpool Publishing who has been so supportive in this project and who has been responsible for bringing this book to you.

I also owe a tremendous debt of gratitude to my friend of many years Henry Burger, Adjunct Professor of Medicine at Monash University in Melbourne, and past president of both the International Menopause Society and the Australian Menopause Society, who read the draft of the book and in so doing contributed so much of his time to confirm the accuracy of the contents, and who made many helpful comments in order to ensure that the information was complete.

Among the many other contributors to the development of the book, I would like to thank Jacqui Dufield, Tina Peers, and Viviane Martin who have assisted in providing material during its conception and genesis.

Without the willing help and advice from so many women, friends and colleagues who contributed so much, this book would never have been completed.

Thank you.

BARRY G. WREN

I have known Barry Wren as a clinician, teacher and confidant for many years. Barry had a knowledgeable voice of reason and concern in the early days of recognition of women and menopause, at a time when research and teaching of this subject was not a fashionable specialty. I am grateful to him for offering me the opportunity and the challenge of co-authoring this book with him. His willingness to allow a peeling back of the hard science to reveal the essence of what needed to be said for and on behalf of women has enabled this book to be written.

I am indebted to the confidences of the many trusting women with whom I have worked in my professional life as a child and family health practitioner, and also to my many friends who have shared the stories of their journeys through their middle years.

I thank Lisa Hanrahan of Rockpool Publishing for believing in this book and I also thank Jody Lee, who has contributed to it as its editor.

I acknowledge the men of my family who have listened in bewilderment to my explanation of the book's content. When they glazed over I knew I had a lot more work to do to present the nature of a woman.

MARGARET STEPHENSON MEERE

Index

About the authors

DR BARRY WREN AM, MD, MBBS, MHP Ed., FRANZCOG, FRCOG

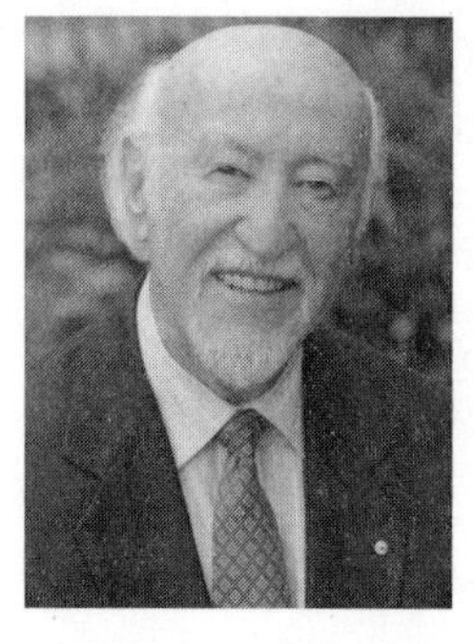

Barry grew up on his father's sheep station in the mid-west of New South Wales and had his early schooling by correspondence. He was awarded a Commonwealth Scholarship to Sydney University and on graduating in 1955, married and began his postgraduate career. His initial research and work as an obstetrician and gynaecologist took him to Western Australia, the United Kingdom and Nigeria before returning to Australia in 1964 where he became Associate Professor in Obstetrics and Gynaecology at the University of NSW. He was always interested in the endocrine health of women and became a founding member of the International Menopause Society in 1976. In the early 1980's he organised meetings of those Australian doctors interested in the health and management of post-menopausal women and began the Australian Menopause Society, becoming its first President in 1988.

He has written many papers and a number of textbooks for students and medical practitioners as well as educational books for women.

In 1997, he was awarded the Australian Menopause Society Medal of Distinction and in 1999 the Australian Government recognised his service to the health of women by awarding him Member of the Order of Australia.

He is married with three sons.

MARGARET STEPHENSON MEERE BA BHSc (Nurs.) RN RM

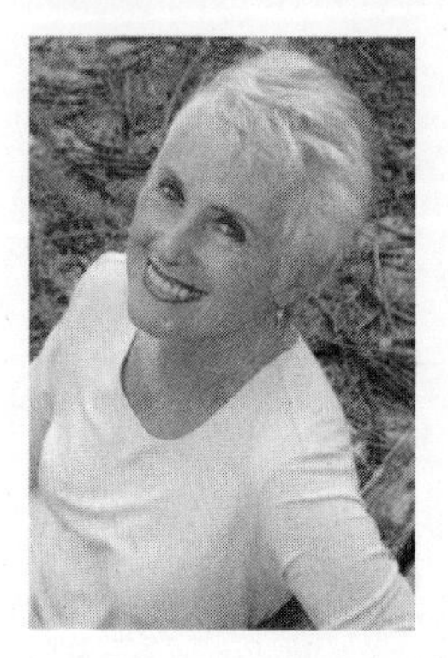

Margaret is a child and family health nurse practitioner.

A qualified nurse/midwife with working experience in both Australia and the United Kingdom, she realised in the 1980s that primary healthcare and education are major contributors to a positive and healthy life experience. She studied Human Bioscience and History to complete her BA and is the author of two books, *Baby's First 100 Days* and *The Child Within the Lotus.*

After living and working in Sydney, Margaret now spends most of her time by a beach on the mid north coast of New South Wales. She is the mother of four sons.